Supporting Learning in Nursing Practice

Nurse Education in Practice Series

Supporting Learning in Nursing Practice: A Guide for Practitioners
Edited by Sally Glen and Pam Parker

Multi-professional Learning for Nurses: Breaking the boundaries
Edited by Sally Glen and Tony Leiba

Problem-based Learning in Nursing: A new model for a new context?
Edited by Sally Glen and Kay Wilkie

Clinical Skills in Nursing: The return of the practical room?
Edited by Maggie Nicol and Sally Glen

Nurse Education in Practice Series
Series Standing Order
ISBN 0–333–98590–7
(outside North America only)

You can receive future titles in this series as they are published by placing a standing order. Please contact your bookseller or, in the case of difficulty, write to us at the address below with your name and address, the title of the series and the ISBN quoted above.

Customer Services Department, Macmillan Distribution Ltd
Houndmills, Basingstoke, Hampshire RG21 6XS, England

Lindsay McClie (signature)

Supporting Learning in Nursing Practice

A guide for practitioners

Edited by

Sally Glen
and
Pam Parker

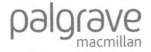

First published 2003 by
PALGRAVE MACMILLAN
Houndmills, Basingstoke, Hampshire RG21 6XS and
175 Fifth Avenue, New York, N.Y. 10010
Companies and representatives throughout the world

PALGRAVE MACMILLAN is the global academic imprint of the Palgrave
Macmillan division of St. Martin's Press, LLC and of Palgrave Macmillan
Ltd. Macmillan® is a registered trademark in the United States, United
Kingdom and other countries. Palgrave is a registered trademark in the
European Union and other countries.

ISBN 1–4039–0292–5

This book is printed on paper suitable for recycling and made from
fully managed and sustained forest sources.

A catalogue record for this book is available from the British Library.

10   9   8   7   6   5   4   3   2   1
12   11   10   09   08   07   06   05   04   03

Typeset by Cambrian Typesetters, Frimley, Surrey

Printed in China

Contents

List of Figures

List of Tables

List of Contributors

Liz Aston RN, RCNT, RNT BSc (open), MRes (Nursing)
Health Lecturer, Practice Learning Team Co-ordinator, School of Nursing, Nottingham University.

Patricia Cronin RN, BSc (Hons) Nursing & Education, MSc Nursing, DipN (Lond) RNT
Senior Lecturer in Nursing St Bartholomew School of Nursing and Midwifery, City University, London.

Professor Lois Crooke RN, RM, MTD, BEd MA (Education) ILT
Pro Vice-Chancellor/Dean Faculty of Health and Human Sciences, Thames Valley University.

Peter Curtis RN, Dip N (Lon), RNT, RCNT, MN
Dean of Clinical Practice in the Wolfson Institute of Thames Valley University.

Val Dimmock MA (Ed) BSc (Nursing) RGN RNT DPSN Cert Ed
Lecturer in Practice St Bartholomew School of Nursing and Midwifery, City University, London.

Chris Ely RN, RM, MSc Continuing ed and training, BA Social Sciences, Cert Ed
Lecturer in Practice St Bartholomew School of Nursing and Midwifery, City University, London.

Sally Glen
Professor of Nursing Education & Dean St Bartholomew's School of Nursing and Midwifery, City University, London.

Diane Lear MA Ed, Cert Ed F.E. RGN, SCM, RCNT, RNT
Lecturer in Education, Course Leader Preparation for Mentorship: St Bartholomew School of Nursing and Midwifery, City University, London.

Maggie Mallik MPhil, BSc (Hons) Nursing Studies, PG Cert Ed, DipN (London) RN
Associate Nurse Executive – Clinical Education, Directorate of Nursing, Salisbury Health Care Trust and Assistant Head of Practice Education, Institute of Health and Community Studies (IHCS) Bournemouth University.

Pam Parker MA (Ed), BA (Hons) Nursing and Education RGN RNT
Senior Lecturer Educational Developments St Bartholomew's School of Nursing and Midwifery, City University, London.

Scott Reeves MSc BSc PGCE
Research Fellow, St Bartholomew School of Nursing and Midwifery City University London & Senior Research Fellow, Queen Mary University of London.

Philippa Sully MSc, RN, RM, RHV, Cert Ed, RNT, FP Cert, CC Relate
Senior Lecturer in Interprofessional Practice St Bartholomew School of Nursing and Midwifery, City University, London.

Gail Thomas RN, RM, ADM, PGCEA, MSc
Dean of Nursing and Midwifery Faculty of Health and Human Sciences, Thames Valley University.

Preface

Supporting Learning in Nursing Practice: A Guide for Practitioners focuses on, as the title suggests, supporting learning in practice. The book is aimed primarily at practitioners who support a range of learners undertaking nurse education programmes. However, many aspects of this book may provide guidance to practitioners from other health and social care professions. *Supporting Learning in Nursing Practice* aims to give some worked examples and practical advice on some of the key issues facing nurse education in this area.

In the United Kingdom (UK) practice-based learning in nursing has long been valued and considered to be of equal importance to institution based learning. The value of a long history of experience in this area should not be underestimated. Chapter 1 outlines a brief history of practice-based learning in nursing in the UK. Three distinct models of nurse eduction are identified are critiqued: pre-1989: apprentice-type model; the 1990s supernumerary model and post-2000: a new model of nurse education.

Chapter 2 continues to examine in more depth issues raised in Chapter 1 related to partnership working to ensure the ongoing quality enhancement of placements as learning environments. Chapter 2 identifies factors that can promote effective learning in practice, along with appropriate learning and teaching strategies. The student's role in practice is explored, alongside the preparation and role of mentors. The chapter concludes with a brief discussion of the link lecturer's role and identifies future strategies that may further enhance practice experience for students.

Chapter 3 further develops this theme of partnership working to ensure the ongoing quality enhancement of placements as learning environments. This chapter describes a practical application of the concept of 'organizational learning' in the context of delivering pre- and post-registration nurse education. The practical application of this concept constitutes a large-scale change which, when successfully implemented, will have far-reaching effects. The chapter starts by setting the contextual scene for this development. It then goes on to explore the theoretical underpinning and concludes by outlining the implications for learning and teaching.

The emphasis of the book then shifts to focus on more specific current key issues in practice-based learning. Problem-based/enquiry-based learning is becoming increasingly popular as a learning and teaching strategy that facilitates the integration of theory and practice and the practical application of formal knowledge.

Chapter 4 reviews how enquiry-based learning (EBL) has evolved from problem-based learning (PBL) and is a method of learning that has been adapted to fulfil the needs of a nursing curriculum in the twenty-first century. This chapter describes an innovative worked example of the application of enquiry-based learning in the practice area.

Chapter 5 explores the premise that the practice of nursing is essentially about effective professional relationships between nurses, those they care for, their peers and colleagues in different professions, and managers. However, the ways in which we learn to make these relationships as practitioners are not necessarily easily explored in the day-to-day supervision of students in practice. This chapter aims to explore some of the skills that nurses who teach in practice might find appropriate to enabling those they supervise to reflect upon and develop their capacities to make effective professional relationships.

The first five chapters in this book therefore discuss a range of activities to support learning in practice and some of the issues associated with the different relationships that support these activities. Chapter 6 brings some of these issues together by focusing on the assessment of learning in practice. This chapter provides an overview of fundamental issues, such as: the reasons practice is assessed and what to assess; and the tools and activities used to assess practice and who should do it. It also provides some practical advice for undertaking the assessment of learning in practice. The three final chapters look to the future.

Chapter 7 builds on one of the themes developed in Chapters 1 and 2 – the need for students to gain insight into the interprofessional team and all the participants' roles. This chapter aims to offer an insight into a range of approaches that can be used by individuals involved in practice-based interprofessional education. The chapter focuses on four factors that help shape this activity: planning processes; learning methods; assessment strategies; and facilitator preparation. To help illuminate the significance of these factors, the chapter discusses the literature in this area and the authors' experience of evaluating practice-based interprofessional education.

Chapter 8 begins by clarifying the nature of practice learning and suggests that the model of 'cognitive apprenticeship' best describes the current role of student nurses in health and social care placements in the UK, with a belief in the 'cognitive apprenticeship' model of practice learning. This chapter suggests that the role of the lecturer/practice educator is not primarily one of providing discrete teaching activities but the much broader role of facilitator of learning and of developing the learning environment. The chapter concludes by offering a number of 'strategies for success'.

The final chapter looks towards the next decade of practice-based learning and proposes a new paradigm for practice education. The earlier chapters have all demonstrated that the problems associated with a culture of practice education by default (unavailability of physical and human resources and few collaborative structures) have, since the late 1990s, been defined and redefined. It is now time to move on. This will require the following: new models of partnership between educators and practising professionals; the development of academic/practice career pathways; a new model of practice education; and the generation of research-based evidence and scholarship that informs policy development and best practice.

1

Practice-based Learning: The Changing Context

Sally Glen

Introduction

In the United Kingdom (UK) nursing practice-based learning has long been valued and considered to be of equal importance to institution-based learning (Burns and Glen, 2000). The value of a long history of experience in this area should not be underestimated. This chapter outlines a brief history of practice-based learning in nursing.

Pre-1989: apprentice-type model

Until 1989, Registered General Nurse programmes were based on an apprentice-type model with much reliance upon experience gained in the clinical setting (traditionally the hospital) as a means of acquiring knowledge and skills. The combination of theoretical periods with associated practical experience, characterized by the pre-1989 training model, had much to commend it. Students learnt quickly, and became more confident, from observing role models practising skills in clinical areas rather than in a classroom. However, the apprentice-type model assumed structured supervision with time for reflection, and not merely exposure to a clinical area (Studdy *et al.*, 1994). It also relied heavily on the assumption that all clinical areas were staffed by highly competent and motivated staff who felt confident enough and had enough time to pass on their skills to student nurses. The adequacy of the apprentice-type model, with its assumption that qualified nurses would teach and supervise student nurses, has been questioned (Orton, 1981; Gott, 1983; Reid, 1985). The emphasis was upon the performance of activities with,

1

as suggested little time for reflection, undermining the potential for learning (Chapman, 1980; UKCC, 1986; Greenwood, 1993).

Traditional nurse education has also been described and characterized by rigidly prescribed nursing curricula, preconceived ideas about the way in which students learnt and were taught, and the repression of creativity (de Tornyay, 1990). It has been asserted that traditionally trained nurses, once qualified, failed to exhibit patient-oriented critical thinking and were not capable of adequate decision making in practice (Heliker, 1994). However, traditional nurse training, based on an apprentice-type model, did produce, at the point of registration, a nurse who had already acquired considerable experience as a member of the nursing workforce and was already perceived by other staff as skilled and experienced. For example, in spite of exhortations to the contrary, students often carried out skilled nursing procedures without supervision and were often left in charge of wards under the nominal supervision of a registered nurse in another part of the hospital. At the same time the role of a staff nurse, whether newly qualified or not, was to manage the work carried out mainly by students rather than to undertake the nursing care herself. The undesirability of this situation, including the paradox that as soon as students became qualified to nurse they ceased to do so in favour of supervising others, was one of the main driving forces for the introduction of the revised pre-registration programmes (Project 2000).

Before the introduction of Project 2000 in 1989 (UKCC, 1986) there were two grades of teacher (Gerrish, 1992): nurse tutors, whose primary responsibility was to teach theory in the classroom, and the clinical teacher, who taught clinical nursing in the practice setting. Clinical teachers covered specific areas/specialities whilst others worked with students across specialities. The nurse tutors also had a clinical role as 'liaison' between service and education, which largely involved information exchange. The roles of the two grades were not always distinct and there was a range of local arrangements, influenced by the individual college of nursing's philosophy and its relationship with relevant clinical areas (Baillie, 1994).

The 1990s: supernumerary model

The first Diploma of Nursing in higher education courses in England began in September 1989. A framework known as Project 2000 (UKCC, 1986) had been established for nurse education which was undoubtedly a radical departure in that it located nursing education firmly within 'higher education'. The introduction of the Diploma of Nursing in higher education courses meant that nursing pre-registration programmes offered students professional registration but also located nursing education completely within the higher education system.

The diploma curriculum structure led to an increased emphasis on health promotion and the prevention of illness. There was a focus on teaching students from a 'wellness' model, thus limiting the students' experiences in the acute setting. There was also a dramatic increase in time spent studying subjects such as the biological sciences, psychology, sociology and health policy. This in turn led to a significant reduction in the time students spent on acquiring psychomotor skills in the classroom. Consequently, a high proportion of students were expected to master what many would argue are essential nursing skills, such as hand washing, bed bathing, temperature, pulse and blood pressure monitoring, and numerous aseptic procedures, while on placements. Students simultaneously gained experience in a wide variety of care settings. They therefore spent less time in the hospital ward setting where nurses traditionally developed and practised skills (Studdy *et al.*, 1994). Furthermore, on qualifying, many students chose to work in an acute setting where patients are anything but 'well' and have complex needs.

The 1990s: from nurse teacher to lecturer in nursing

The amalgamation of colleges of nursing and midwifery and their subsequent transfer into higher education, together with the need for individuals to undertake degree-level study and higher, created a very stressful period for nurse teachers. In addition, the United Kingdom Central Council (UKCC, 1986) encouraged the establishment of only one grade of teacher and at the same time suggested that a teaching presence in the clinical settings was necessary for the successful development of Project 2000 practitioners. The UKCC's (1986) view was that nurse teachers should be able to demonstrate advanced theoretical and clinical knowledge. The Department of Health's *Strategy for Nursing* (1989) provided support for this by stating the nurse teachers should be credible in the area of practice they teach. The strategy also stipulated that they should be linked to clinical areas. The English National Board (ENB, 1989) similarly indicated that nurse teachers should retain their clinical competence and be able to teach in the classroom and in practice settings.

Crotty and Butterworth (1992) acknowledged the complexity of the nurse teacher's role and described the requirements as: a nurse, a teacher, a graduate in a specialist subject and both clinically and educationally credible. It is not surprising that, amidst these developments, the need for nurse teachers to develop a role in the clinical area as the clinical teacher numbers diminished was afforded minimal importance by most nurse teachers and their managers. This caused serious concern because, although the conflicts of meeting the demands of the clinical teaching role were documented in such a way as to lead to the recommendation to discontinue preparation for the role (Kirkwood, 1979; Clifford, 1993), there had been no apparent nationwide effort to provide the substitute for the aspects of the role that were positively rated. For example, Gott (1983) and Reid (1985) noted the positive benefits of the clinical teaching role in contributing towards a good learning environment. Mallik and Aston (Chapter 8) note that there was relatively little systematic study completed on the impact or effectiveness of the clinical teacher post apart from the descriptive work completed by Kirkwood (1979), Robertson (1987) and Martin (1989). There was, and is, no tradition of a clinical academic career in nursing. Entering a career as a nurse educator has demanded that individuals give up the clinical career in which they have become expert and experienced. Medicine and dentistry, of course, have a long history of university-based education and their teaching in the clinical areas is supported by an identified funding stream (Committee of Vice-Chancellors and Principals (CVCP), 1997, see also Chapter 9).

The 1990s: trained nurse – clinician, manager and educator

During the 1990s several key national documents outlined the changing context of healthcare delivery, for example: *A Vision for the Future – The Nursing, Midwifery and Health Visiting Contribution to Health and Healthcare* (DOH, 1993); *Challenges for Nursing and Midwifery Education in the 21st Century – The Heathrow Debate* (DOH, 1994); and *The National Health Service – A Service With Ambition* (DOH, 1996). All these policy documents identified factors that have had an influence on the type and numbers of nurses needed, and on the knowledge, skills and attitudes they required to meet the health needs of the population. Far-reaching changes to both healthcare needs and service provision also made it increasingly difficult for students to develop skills through repetition. These changes included a decline in the number of acute hospital beds, an increased emphasis upon day surgery, a move towards intermediate and home care, coupled with a major shift of resources into community care provision. These factors have led to an increasingly finite, specialized, often unpredictable, clinical resource, with far sicker patients who should not be subjected to the practice of the novice (Studdy *et al.*, 1994).

Consideration must also be given to the NHS reforms which have resulted in clinical staff balancing conflicting demands in their management, clinical and educational roles. Many areas saw a reduction in the number of permanent qualified staff, whilst the development of healthcare assistant training meant an increased supervisory and assessment role. The qualified nurses' role, in terms of supervising diploma students, was reported to have been undermined by inadequate initial preparation of trained staff during the development and implementation phase of Project 2000 (Jowett and Walton, 1995). Trained nurses also expressed concern about: finding enough qualified staff to act as supervisors; the heavy burden of supervision given the students:staff ratios; and the heightened demands in terms of time and responsibility of teaching and supervising students undertaking the Common Foundation Programme (CFP) who allegedly possessed not even basic practical nursing skills (Bedford *et al.*, 1993; Elkan and Robinson, 1995). Jowett and Walton (1995), in a longitudinal study of the process of implementing 'Project 2000' programmes in six of the thirteen first-round demonstration districts, found that named mentors played a limited role in ensuring that a student's placement experience was educationally sound.

The introduction of the education-led diploma programmes had undoubtedly been successful in increasing the academic status of nursing. However, higher cognitive skills, combined with more varied and less predictable clinical experience, had led to a perceived lack of skills and confidence on the part of newly qualified student nurses.

The 1990s: newly qualified diplomates: strengths and concerns

By the mid-1990s a discourse was emerging that was beginning to raise questions about the clinical competence of newly qualified diplomates (Glen and Clark, 1999). Amongst Project 2000 diplomates interviewed by Runciman *et al.* (1998), ($n = 1,349$) 74 per cent felt that more practical skills in the university would have improved their preparation and 54 per cent felt that more assessment of practice would have been helpful. Elkan and Robinson (1995), in their research into the implementation of Project 2000, found that the first students to emerge from these courses felt awkward and ill at ease during their early placements. The students interviewed attributed this to a lack of practice competence. The Macleod Clark *et al.* (1996) study also seemed to confirm the picture of strengths and concerns; in addition to a perceived lack of skills, practice experience and confidence and need for preceptorship (of up to one year), there appeared to be concerns about newly qualified nurses' attitudes, possibly limited due to supernumerary status. The change to supernumerary status did not, of course, necessarily change people's expectations of newly qualified nurses.

The expectations and attitudes of traditionally trained nurses were also complex. For example, in a survey of qualified nurses in the Western Isles Health Board ($n = 179$l – a 51 per cent response rate) Cuthbertson (1996) found that the commonly held view that Project 2000 nurses were not well prepared, particularly in relation to having enough practical skills, was based on faulty knowledge about the education programmes. Hickey (1996) also reported concern about a lack of emphasis on practical skills, although she suggests that opinions may have been formed on the basis of working with students in the early Common Foundation Programme (CFP) period. It also seemed that some traditionally trained nurses perceived themselves as likely to be disadvantaged in the labour market on the assumption that Project 2000 nurses would increasingly be favoured.

The *Fitness for Purpose* report (Luker *et al.*, 1996), commissioned by the DOH, found that managers regarded diplomates as articulate, questioning, enthusiastic, flexible in approach and willing to challenge. There was evidence of satisfactory cognitive abilities, but once again a degree of lack of confidence in clinical competence than might have been expected on first taking up a staff nurse post. Managers' expectations regarding skills acquisition were also not always realized, particularly in relation to 'core' skills, such as drug administration. Diplomates were allegedly very quick to acquire these skills once qualified. Managers in the community felt that diplomates had excellent written and verbal skills, although there was some disagreement about levels of interpersonal skills development and about abilities of newly qualified diplomates to take up posts in the community immediately. It was felt, however, that diplomates were better prepared than traditionally trained nurses to work in the community (Runciman *et al.*, 1998).

The emergence of new roles such as that of healthcare assistant, and the extension of the scope and range of practice of experienced nurses, was also thought to be having an effect on the newly qualified staff nurse, to the extent that there was some difficulty in defining clearly the role of the D grade nurse. Luker *et al.* (1996, p. 69) suggests that for managers:

it was almost as if by introducing such new roles at the bottom end of the scale, all other roles above this, including the D grade, had shifted upwards a notch. Thus they had lost the unskilled tasks at the bottom and gained the extended role at the top. Even if some (managers) argued that the diplomates didn't even have the basic skills, others were able to provide evidence that they didn't need them, but that they (new staff nurses) did have the more sophisticated knowledge and skills which had become valued in the D grade role.

Murray (1996) also advises caution in using the results of Project 2000 studies: first, in relation to how adequately all four branches' views are represented; second, education programmes are not static, that both small and large changes tend to be introduced year on year in response to monitoring and quality assurance processes (Runciman *et al.*, 1998); and third, in relation to the changing context of nursing care which affects both education and practice. However, the principles of the original Project 2000 proposal, *A New Preparation for Practice* (UKCC, 1986), were to produce practitioners able to contribute to planning, assessing and developing services, particularly in primary care settings, with a readiness to face change. The UKCC Commission for Nursing and Midwifery Education (UKCC, 1999) concluded that the principles were, to some extent, weakened on implementation because of ongoing developments in the health services and in education.

The implementation of Project 2000, with its higher theoretical demands on students and teachers, many of whom were unprepared for the role (Davies *et al.*, 1996), has also created the need to re-evaluate, once again, the clinical role of the nurse teacher (Lee, 1996). Should they become a visitor, performing a liaison function, should they perform a clinical teaching function or be a role model for clinical practice?

Post-2000: a new model of nurse education

Many commentators also believed by the end of the 1990s that pre-registration education programmes had too much theory and too little practice, particularly during the early stages (Hislop *et al.*, 1996). It could also be argued that there was insufficient attention to the integration of theory and practice in the real world. This had led to the inclusion of inappropriate or irrelevant material within the curriculum.

In July 1999 the Department of Health published the nursing strategy *Making a Difference*. This strategy document launched proposals for a new model of nurse education and a stronger role for the NHS in the management of pre-registration nursing education. *Making a Difference* (DOH, 1999) notes a loss of a link between students and their 'home' hospital, making it more difficult to recruit and retain staff. More pertinently, the importance of practice placements in the education of healthcare professionals was emphasized as part of the Department of Health's drive to modernize the NHS. *Making a Difference* suggests that the placements needed to be of higher quality, accompanied by enhanced teacher support to help students gain better practical skills (p. 23). The announcement in the same document of 6000 additional training places to be made available over the following three years created both a challenge and an opportunity to address the need for more quality clinical placements in both primary and secondary care (p. 18).

From September 2000 the *Fitness for Practice* (UKCC, 1999) model of nurse education was implemented in 16 partnership sites. This model introduced more flexibility in nurse education with 'stepping on and off points'. In addition, standards required for registration as a nurse were constructed in terms of outcomes for theory and practice. Consequently there are common outcomes for the end of year one of the pre-registration programme, and competencies for the end of year three of the programme (UKCC, 2000). In particular, these reforms, through Accreditation of Prior Learning and Experience (AP(E)L), mean that non-professional staff are able to access professional education utilizing previous knowledge and experience. For example, through the attainment of National Vocational Qualification (NVQ) Level 3, non-professional staff are able to fast-track into nurse education programmes. New cadet schemes also operated from September 2000. These schemes offer a vocational pathway into nurse education as they result in the award of vocational qualifications.

The implementation of *Fitness for Practice* (UKCC, 1999) has also created opportunities for nurse educators to rekindle their clinical practice skills and enabled an appropriate sharing of responsibility for students' clinical learning between higher education institutes (HEIs) and the NHS Learning and exposure to good role models in placements has long been recognized as being more influential than learning and role models within HEIs. Students' practice experience is now widely acknowledged as being one of the most important facets of their educational preparation in health and social care. As Napthine (1996), quoted in Nolan (1998), writes: 'The quality of nursing education is dependent upon the quality of students' clinical experience. Clinical placement experience is central to the development of nursing practical skills' (p. 623).

The access and availability of quality placements was therefore a theme running through many policy documents between 1999 and 2002. The UKCC Commission for Nursing and Midwifery Education Report, *Fitness for Practice* (UKCC, 1999), suggests that: 'practice placements should be designed to achieve agreed outcomes which benefit student learning and provide experience of the full 24 hour per day and seven day per week nature of health care' (p. 41).

The CVCP and NHS Executive's and *Partnership Statement* (CVCP and NHS Executive, 1999) requires that placement opportunities should be of good quality, provide relevant learning, give adequate support to students and have jointly agreed learning outcomes. The importance of clinical experience was also stressed in *A Health Service Of All The Talents: Developing the NHS Workforce* (DOH, 2000a), which places clear responsibility on employers and the Workforce Development Confederations to establish good-quality practice placements. In January 2001 the DOH/English National Board (ENB) document, *Placements in Focus: Guidance for Education in Practice for Health Care Professions*, emphasized that it is widely acknowledged that students' practice experience is one of the most important facets of their educational preparation in health and social care. This document also emphasizes that enhancing the quality and innovative development of practice placements is an integral part of the Government's modernization agenda (DOH/ENB, 2001). In July 2001 the Quality Assurance Agency (QAA) issued the *Code of Practice for the Assurance of Academic Quality and Standards in Higher Education: Placement Learning (Section 9)*. This document also stresses the need for a partnership between the NHS and HEIs.

Educating and training the future health professional workforce for England (report by the Comptroller and Auditor General HC 277, Session 2000-2001: 1 March 2001) noted: 'The availability of practice placements is one of the key factors in determining the number of students that can be trained and influences the quality of outcomes' (p. 2, Box A). Moreover, the *Workforce Development Confederations' Guidance* (DOH, 2000b) noted: 'Confederations will promote the development of local quality assurance and performance programmes by provision and maintenance of high quality placements, practice and experience' (para. 12), and elsewhere the report recommends: 'Work with [i.e. the Workforce Development Confederations' work with] higher education institutions to develop and implement joint strategies to address the problems in arranging good quality practice placements, identifying alternative suitable placements in the NHS and the wider health economy' (p. 5). The

Workforce Development Confederations (WDCs) were established with the explicit directive to work in partnership with HEIs, appoint HEI representatives to executive boards and take joint responsibility with HEIs for the provision of placements. For example, 'The Confederations will have responsibility for practice placements for all students on N.H.S. and HEFCE funded health care training programmes' (DOH, 2002, para. 25).

The *Human Resources Performance Framework* (NHS Executive, 2001) also emphasizes the need for joint strategies to develop and enhance placement quality and capacity. The challenges for both HEIs and the NHS in relation to both enhancing the quality and capacity of practice placements are:

- to enhance placement quality and capacity to meet additional training placements,
- to identify and develop innovative placements both with the NHS and by looking at the opportunities within the voluntary and independent sectors,
- to establish a 'managed system' to facilitate a working partnership between HEIs, WDCs, the NHS and the independent sector and between professions with a named person responsible, and
- more formalized preparation, support and updating of supervisors, assessors and mentors to provide confident and competent role models.

In April 2002 the Department of Health and the Higher Education Funding Council for England announced a *Statement of Strategic Alliance for Health and Social Care* (DOH, 2000c). In the foreword it states: 'The Strategic Alliance further strengthens the commitment of both organisations to partnership working, providing the framework for building upon existing liaison, consultation and representation ... The Alliance should be seen as providing the context for a wider set of health and education sector partnerships.' A range of initiatives within the partnership arrangements between HEIs, WDCs and Trusts is therefore required to increase the level of support and supervision for students gaining practice experience. The central issue, which must be of concern, is the extent to which this new expressed policy commitment to partnership translates into reality at the many strategic and operational interfaces between the NHS and HEIs.

Conclusion

The present culture of 'clinical education by default', unavailability of mentors and general lack of formal collaborative structures between education and service institutions cannot sustain the complex demands, expectations and pace of the clinical context and the evolution of nursing practice. The key challenge is undoubtedly to ensure that all students have access to quality learning experiences with mentors and supervisors who are prepared to meet the healthcare challenges of the twenty-first century. This issue is taken up again in the final chapter of this book.

References

Baillie, L, (1994) Nurse Teachers Feeling About Participating In Clinical Practice: An exploratory study, *Journal of Advanced Nursing*, **20**, 150–9.

Bedford, H, Phillips, T, Robinson, J and Schostak, J (1993) *Assessing Competencies in Nursing and Midwifery Education and Training (Ace Report)*. London: English National Board.

Burns, I, and Glen, S (2000) An Educational Model for Preparation for Practice. In Glen, S and Wilkie, K (eds), *Problem-Based Learning in Nursing: A New Model for A New Context*, Basingstoke: Macmillan Press – now Palgrave Macmillan.

Chapman, C (1980) The Learner as Worker: Issues in Nurse Education, *Medical Teacher*, **2**(5), 241–4.

Clifford, C (1993) The Clinical Role of The Nurse Teacher in the UK, *Journal of Advanced Nursing* **18**, 281–9.

Committee of Vice-Chancellors and Principals (1997) *Clinical Academic Careers: Report of An Independent Task Force*. Chaired by Professor Rex Richard.

Committee of Vice-Chancellors and Principals and NHS Executive (1999) *Partnership Statement*.

Comptroller and Auditor General (2001) *Educating and training the future health professional workforce for England*, HC 277 Session 2000–2001.

Crotty, M, and Butterworth, T (1992) The Emerging Role of the Nurse Teacher in Project 2000 Programmes in England: A Literature Review, *Journal of Advanced Nursing*, **17**, 1377–87.

Cuthbertson, P (1996) Attitudes to Project 2000: a survey of qualified nurses, *Nursing Standard*, **11**(11), 38–41.

Davies, S, White, E, Riley, E and Twinn, S (1996) How can Nurse Teachers be More Effective in Practice Settings? *Nurse Education Today*, **16**, 19–27.

Department of Health (1989) Strategy for Nursing. London: HMSO.

Department of Health (1993) *A Vision for the Future – The Nursing, Midwifery and Health Visiting Contribution to Health and Healthcare*. London: HMSO.

Department of Health (1994) *Challenges for Nursing and Midwifery Education in the Twenty-First Century – the Heathrow Debate*. London: HMSO.

Department of Health (1996) *The National Health Service – A Service with Ambition*, London: HMSO.

Department of Health (1999) *Making a Difference: Strengthening the Nursing, Midwifery and Health Visiting Contribution to Health and Healthcare.* London: DOH.

Department of Health (2000a) *Consultative Document: A Health Service Of All The Talents: Developing the NHS Workforce.* London: DOH.

Department of Health (2000b) *Workforce Development Confederations' Guidance.* London: DOH.

Department of Health and the Higher Education Funding Council for England (2000c) *Statement of Strategic Alliance for Health and Social Care.* London: DOH.

Department of Health/English National Board (2001) *Placements in Focus: Guidance for Education in Practice for Health Care Professions.* London: DOH/ENB.

Department of Health (2002) *Workforce Development Confederations' Functions, Accountabilities and Working Relationships.* London: DOH.

De Tornyay, R (1990) The Curriculum Revolution, *Journal of Nursing Education*, **29**, 292–4.

Elkan, R and Robinson, J (1995) Project 2000: a review of published research, *Journal of Advanced Nursing*, **22**, 386–92.

English National Board (1989) *Preparation of Teachers, Practitioners, Mentors and Supervisors. In the Context of Project 2000.* Consultative Paper. London: ENB.

Gerrish, K (1992) The Nurse Teacher's Role In The Practice Setting, *Nurse Education Today*, **12**, 227–32.

Glen, S and Clark, A (1999) Nurse Education: a skill mix for the future, *Nurse Education Today*, **19**, 12–19.

Gott, M (1983) The Preparation of the Student for Learning in the Clinical Setting. In Davies, B D (ed.), *Research into Nurse Education.* Beckenham, Kent: Croom Helm.

Greenwood, J (1993) *Reflective Practice: A critique of the work of Argyris and Schon, Journal of Advanced Nursing*, **18**, 1183–7.

Heliker, D (1994) Meeting the Challenge of the Curriculum Revolution: Problem Based Learning in Nurse Education, *Journal of Nursing Education*, **33**, 457.

Hickey, G (1996) The Challenge of Change in Nurse Education: Traditionally Trained Nurses' Perception of Project 2000, *Nurse Education Today*, **16**, 389–96.

Hislop, S, Inglis, B, Cope, P, Stoddart, B and McIntosh, C (1996) Situating Theory in Practice: Student Views of Theory – Practice in Project 2000 Nursing Programmes, *Journal of Advanced Nursing*, **23**, 171–7.

Jowett, S and Walton, I (1995*) Challenges and Changes. Nurse Education: A Study of the Implementation of Project 2000.* London: NFER.

Kirkwood, L, (1979) The Clinical Teacher, Occasional Paper, *Nursing Times*, **75**(12), 59–61.

Lee, D T F (1996) The Clinical Role of the Nurse Teacher: A review of the dispute, *Journal of Advanced Nursing*, **23**, 1127–1134.

Luker, K, Carlisle, C, Riley, E *et al.* (1996) Project 2000, *Fitness for Purpose Report to the Department of Health.* London: DOH.

Macleod Clark, J, Maben, J and Jones, K (1996) *Project 2000: perceptions of the philosophical practice of nursing.* London: English National Board for Nursing, Midwifery and Health Visiting.

Martin, L (1989) *Clinical Education in Perspective.* London: Royal College of Nursing.

Murray, C (1996) ENB report on Project 2000: is there cause to celebrate?, *British Journal of Nursing,* **5**(13), 776.

Napthine, R (1996) Clinical Education: A System Under Pressure, *Australian Nursing Journal,* **3**(9), 20–24.

National Health Services Executive (2001) *Human Resources Performance Framework.* Leeds: NHS Executive.

Nolan, C A (1998) Learning On Clinical Placements: The Experience of Six Australian Student Nurses, *Nurse Education Today,* **18**(8) L622–8.

Orton A (1981) *Ward Learning Climate: A Study of the Role of the Ward Sister in Relation to Student Nurse Learning on the Ward,* London: RCN.

Quality Assurance Agency (QAA) *Code of Practice for the Assurance of Academic Quality and Standards in Higher Education: Placement Learning (Section 9).* Bristol: QAA.

Reid, N G (1985) *Wards in Chancery.* London: RCN.

Robertson, C M (1987) *A Very Special Form of Teaching.* London: RCN.

Runciman, P, Dewar, B and Goulbourne A (1998) *Project 2000 in Scotland: Employers' Needs and the Skills of Newly Qualified Project 2000 Staff Nurses.* Edinburgh: Queen Margaret College.

Studdy, S J, Nicol M and Fox-Hiley, H D (1994) Teaching and Learning Clinical Skills Part 1 – Development of a Teaching Model and Schedule of Skills Development, *Nurse Education Today,* **14**, 186–93.

UKCC (1986) *A New Preparation for Practice.* London: UKCC.

UKCC (1999) *Fitness for Practice.* The UKCC Commission for Nursing and Midwifery Education, chaired by Sir Leonard Peach. London: UKCC.

UKCC (2000) *Nursing Competencies SN/PW/PO ed/letters n.comp 1012.* London: UKCC.

2

The Practice Learning Experience

Christine Ely and Diane Lear

Introduction

This chapter will continue to examine some of the issues raised in Chapter 1 related to the quality of the practice placement. There will be a discussion of the environment and what factors can promote effective learning, and the learning and teaching strategies that can support it. The students role in practice will also be explored as will the preparation and role of the mentors who support students during their experience. The chapter will conclude with a brief discussion of the link lecturer's role and future actions that may enhance practice experience further.

Promoting effective learning in the practice area

The *Placements in Focus* document stressed that the environment should provide an arena in which students can experience good-quality care and treatment of patients and clients (DOH/ENB, 2001a). This is discussed as being achieved through several actions, which include:

- qualified staff providing good 'role models' for best practice, valuing learning and encouraging reflection;
- students experiencing good leadership in a variety of settings where healthcare is provided;
- students experiencing the positive culture of clinical governance, which is based on evidence-based approaches;
- staff reflecting on practice providing a climate that is proactive and challenging;

- a multiprofessional focus on care, enabling students to observe how all of the staff contribute to the provision of care.

Before allocation of students to an area, specific efforts must be made to consider the kind of learning environment it provides, and required changes must be implemented so that it is able to meet the educational needs of both students and trained staff through an educational audit. As professionals, all nursing staff must be committed to the concept of life-long learning and demonstrate this by meeting the PREP (Post Registration Education and Practice) requirements (UKCC, 1994).

Preparing for the allocation of students should prompt the staff to reappraise their own psychological and physical learning environment. This process enables changes to be initiated that will ensure it is an environment that meets both student and staff needs for proactive, continual development. This is a positive process, which in the past has only received scant attention (Carlisle, 1991), but as Maggs (1996) noted, the presence of an effective continuing professional education facility positively influences recruitment and retention of staff.

Physical learning environment

As all healthcare professionals are encouraged to be lifelong learners (Morton-Cooper and Palmer, 2000), a dedicated/designated teaching or seminar room should be available in all practice areas. Within this area there should be specific resources for student teaching and learning. Equipment used for teaching should be maintained to required safety standards and allowance should be made for this in the practice area budget. The teaching area should have appropriate furniture, ventilation and lighting. Adapted areas, that is, staff rest rooms, patients' day rooms and nursing stations, are not suitable for structured teaching. The designated teaching area may also be used for instructing patients and relatives, thus maximizing the use of this resource. Impressions are important, and a teaching room that is proactively maintained, with current publications and other learning materials, is a clear indication that learning and continuous professional development is valued and an ongoing organized activity. There should be a clearly apparent organisational culture that values learning, noted by Sapienza (1985) cited in Holloway (1991, p. 136), as a 'shared appreciative system'. Learning in practice is a two-way process; specific literature linked to student assessment requirements, and the sharing of knowledge and experience, will encourage students to furnish the practice area with up-to-date research and publications. They should be encouraged to participate in clinical knowledge provision, by sharing ideas on practice issues, facilitated by being given time to visit the library (DOH/ENB, 2001a).

Psychosocial learning environment

The psychosocial element of the learning environment also requires consideration. Quinn (2000) describes it as 'a holistic notion'. Students need to feel valued, and provided with a sense of security and trust, which will enable them to challenge assumptions and ask questions. Students require the freedom to learn, from competent role models, in a stimulating and supportive environment where there are clearly demonstrated links between nursing theory and practice (Nicklin and Kenworthy, 2000). They should feel that their novice or advanced beginner status is acknowledged and that they are recognized as having a need to learn to be, and practise the skills required of, a nurse (Neary, 1997). Students on placement need time to reflect and seek peer support, an activity fostered in the classroom which can be replicated and provided in practice through small-group reflective discussion sessions, or student-led seminars. Participation in these activities, as well as encouragement and support to seek answers in a variety of ways, will reduce students' feelings of isolation, which can be a barrier to learning (Haddock, 1997; Smith and Gray, 2001).

Staff attitudes to the learning programme

It is also important that learners feel that their programme is valid and appropriate as a preparation for professional life. Staff in practice areas may demonstrate negative, dismissive attitudes to the academic, theoretical aspects of the learning programme and they may view it as irrelevant or impractical (Stengelhofen, 1993). Kramer (1974) identified how professional staff, on entering the workplace and by surviving their experience of reality shock, may have done so through maladaptive behaviours. Therefore preparing learners for reality shock may lessen their experience of conflict and the contradictions that occur in practice in a health service that may not always have optimum levels of resources. These issues, if raised before placements begin, prepare learners for practice reality. Discussion and reflection with trained nurses and link lecturers during placement should also enable learners to challenge work practices in a constructive, non-threatening way. Denying learners this opportunity will create a barrier to learning through reflection (Boud and Walker, 1993).

Orientation of students to clinical areas

Students arriving in practice areas would be more prepared if they had some orientation to the area before placement there. As soon as the practice area has been informed of the number, and level of experience, of the students who will be attending their area, a letter of welcome should be sent to each individual. In this way explanation of the area's specialty, shift patterns, and any specific issues/requirements, for example uniform or 'mufti', that should be known can be explained in advance. Just as patients can be confused by scientific language or jargon (Sundeen *et al.*, 1998), students need clarification in regard to terminology used in the area of nursing practice that they will be going to. For totally new experiences, a full glossary of common terms provided in advance will empower the student, and reduce their perceived level of confusion.

When the student begins the placement there should be some formal orientation, which should include the generic issues in Figure 2.1; in addition there are orientation packages, which should include the learner-specific issues outlined in Figure 2.2.

Generic issues

Policies/procedures:
Health & Safety; manual handling; use of medicines;
legal documentation; confidentiality; risk assessment;
use of dangerous substances; resuscitation & fire

Equipment:
Extinguishers; hoists; bathing aids and so on

Geographic:
Area layout; fire exits; link facilities; link departments;
map of community and surrounding area; transport

Personnel:
Multidisciplinary team; community care teams

Figure 2.1   Generic issues for placements

```
┌─────────────────────────────────────────────────────────────────┐
│                     Learner-specific issues                       │
│                                                                   │
│                              HCA                                  │
│                      NVQ level 1, 2 or 3                          │
│                                                                   │
│                       Pre-registration                            │
│           Year 1, 2 & 3 curriculum-specific/personal             │
│                                                                   │
│                 Newly qualified/preceptee                         │
│               Specialty/grade/role/personal                       │
│                                                                   │
│                   Specialist practice                             │
│             Course/module-specific/personal                       │
│                                                                   │
│                    Staff development                              │
│     Role-specific/level-specific/personal academic or practice    │
└─────────────────────────────────────────────────────────────────┘
```

Figure 2.2   Learner-specific issues for placements

The discussion so far has highlighted some of the factors that can affect the learning environment and how these may be enhanced. In conjunction with this there are learning and teaching strategies that can be used to support learning in practice.

Learning and teaching strategies to promote effective learning

Learning in practice should be supported and encouraged through both formal and informal strategies. Students require direction and guidance and should also be encouraged to develop the skill of self-assessment through reflective practice activities.

Formal teaching sessions

A teaching programme that meets both the trained nurses and students' needs should be evident. These are often presented as a rolling programme and trained staff can utilize individual sessions to meet their own developmental needs. Specialist perspectives, for example tissue viability, or dealing with violence in the workplace, may be the remit of a particular staff member as part of their commitment to practice development. Their responsibility is to expand knowledge through the sharing of research findings with the whole team.

Participation in this process should clearly indicate to students that formal instruction is an integral aspect of practice learning, which complements the more informal learning that occurs when discussing, observing and participating with professional staff during all stages of care delivery.

Ideally the formal learning programme should cover a variety of subjects and use various teaching methods. It should be planned following an assessment of learning needs (Panno, 1992). Students should be encouraged to participate fully with senior students who undertake some of the teaching.

Although education is aimed primarily to meet specific local training needs, a broader content can be provided to fulfil both student and trained staff requirements (Shepherd, 1994). The programme should run concurrently with student placement time frames, but allow space and time for evaluation to ensure appropriate content before it is begun. The programme can be effectively evaluated by explicit goal attainment measures (Fleck and Fyffe, 1997). At the beginning of a placement allocation personal learning goals for the individual student, or continuing education goals for permanent staff, can be mutually agreed.

Role model: professional social learning

Trained nurses should ensure that their practice is current, reflective and evidence based. Students should be encouraged to observe and emulate best practice, in a culture that is proactive and encourages behaviours based on professional guidelines (DOH/ENB, 2001a; Oliver and Endersby, 1994). Bandura (1977a), cited in Bahn (2001), highlights that modelling is a powerful medium for the transmission of required values, attitudes, ways of thinking and behaviour patterns.

Learning contracts

Critical analysis can be observed and learnt from a role model, but this is not always sufficient and more direction may be necessary. Learning contracts can be used as a means of promoting the control of learning to be assumed by the individual learner. Central to the use of contract learning is that learners specify their own evaluative criteria and outcomes. This echoes Knowles's (1986), cited in Jarvis (2000), premise that students need to be encouraged to be self-directed. Jarvis (2000) notes that contracts work well in areas where practical learning is required and that they should be mutually generated but encourage the student's autonomy. Knowles (1990), cited in Quinn (2000), sets out eight stages required for the development of a contract:

- Diagnosis of need, where the present level of knowledge/skill is assessed, in relation to the aim for learning achievement, set against the opportunities presented through which learning can be processed.
- Specifying learning objectives, when needs are translated into objectives statements.
- Specifying learning resources and strategies, when a plan is set out for how each objective will be achieved and what resources are required to facilitate this.
- Specifying evidence of accomplishment, when evidence is described that will be produced to indicate successful attainment.
- Specifying how evidence will be validated, when the stated criteria for measurement of set levels of achievement are denoted, whether these are academic or practice based.
- Review the contract with consultants – the initial draft is reviewed with the practice mentor to verify that the aims and outcomes are clear and relevant.
- Implement the contract – adjustments are made as learning progresses.
- Evaluating learning – here the achievement of aims and outcome attainments are verified by the practice mentor.

Use of learning contracts requires the learner to be active within the learning process and is a vital motivating factor. It emphasizes the need for student responsibility for learning, an important factor in lifelong learning (Quinn, 2000; DOH/ENB, 2001a and b).

Informal lectures, seminars and discussions groups

Structured learning will promote feelings of value within learners, knowing that they have been taught (Quinn, 2000). Seminars can encourage students to explore new thinking or practice protocols, in areas that may be new or less familiar to trained staff. Through the dissemination of research findings students can contribute to clinical knowledge, and be empowered by taking the lead in this learning approach. The discussion following a seminar, involving all levels of participants, will enable the learners' value systems and beliefs to be shared, critiqued and confirmed, and give rise to new concepts and ideas, and analysed in the light of practice reality (Nicklin and Kenworthy, 2000).

Discussion Groups can be open forums or directed by the need to explore designated topics. Due to their open, participative nature, such groups encourage the student to freely contribute their views and opinions. These can be solely nursing in focus or multiprofessional. Another aspect of this type of learning forum is the journal club, with a specific aim or focus. These produce learning foci for students similar to seminars.

Demonstration(s)

Trained staff can demystify specialist equipment in use in their area by demonstrating how to use it safely, and by encouraging the learner to practise its use in a controlled situation or way. Clinical skills, both general and specific, can be learnt through the demonstration and rehearsal process, with trained staff demonstrating the skill in totality, then deconstructing this in to its component parts and leading the learner through its reconstruction. The learner should then talk the staff member through the process, receiving constructive feedback on performance. Students can also be aided to learn psychomotor skills with mental rehearsal of the skill to enhance learning (Bowles, 1995). Guidance should be given and opportunities to practise provided till both learner and trained staff become confident with the level of competence demonstrated.

Question and answer sessions

Students can assess their own learning achievement or needs in question and answer sessions, which are, and is a useful strategy to employ at the conclusion of other teaching methods. Self-assessment is a lifelong learning skill, which will facilitate professional development. Pre-registration students are predominantly assessed summatively; however, with the transition to registered practitioner they are expected to be adept in self-assessment. This is a skill requisite for enabling them to meet their continuing professional development needs (Purdy, 1997). It is also a strategy which requires the learner to participate actively in the learning process.

Role-play and simulation

Strategies of role-play and simulation can be utilized to provide learners with a safe mechanism to experience issues such as control and restraint techniques, or sensitive issues such as the breaking of bad news. They are often employed to explore interpersonal issues, and can be a powerful medium for learning but need to be expertly devised, controlled and delivered. The learner is enabled to act out new skills and/or test new concepts, which encourages learning in all domains – cognition, attitudinal and skill based. By practising before performing skills in the client care arena, students can stumble, but through positive, constructive feedback, will remain confident and motivated (Nicklin and Kenworthy, 2000).

Case studies

Staff or students can present a case review that is of current interest. The discussion and dialogue generate a vehicle for the dissemination of best practice, and allow for care packages to be explored and rationalized. Students are enabled to fully examine symptoms, diagnostic indicators and treatment regimens under supervision and guidance from trained professionals. They will also observe how care is evaluated. Whilst all details of the client remain confidential, the student is enabled to witness theory applied to real problems, and relate to and reflect on issues raised.

The patient/client as a visual aid, or model

Reality-based learning requires that patients are included in the overall scheme of practice exposure. It allows a 'hands-on approach' to skill acquisition, and is a vital method for learning (Harding, 1979). However, it must always be approached with caution to avoid some of the legal and ethical pitfalls, for example consent and confidentiality issues (NMC, 2002), which includes the need to seek the permission of the patient.

Patients and their relatives are subject to anxiety arising from ill-health and the need for hospitalization. Their stress may initiate complex responses, demonstrated through a wide range of behaviour, for example extreme gratitude or anger and resentment (Lyth, 1988). Therefore, if the teaching purpose cannot be perceived as appropriate or of direct benefit, or results in inept practice, this may cause an increase in stress for both patient and relatives. The Patient's Charter (DOH, 1996) empowers clients to refuse to be included in the teaching of students, and informed consent should be sought without undue coercion to cooperate. Patients' autonomous status must be maintained and acknowledged.

The involvement of patients in teaching may have positive or negative consequences for them. It could facilitate an increased level of knowledge and understanding of their diagnosis and treatment regimens. It may make them feel that they are interesting, or they may use it as a strategy to prevent feelings of boredom, and therefore value the increased contact time with nursing staff. Negative elements are usually the converse, in that patients may feel excluded if students are not directed to focus their conversations and questions through the patient. They may feel confused if jargon or medical terminology is left unexplained or over-used. They may come to feel that staff are only interested in their condition and not in them as a person, so students should be encouraged to approach patients and to ask them to elucidate their health status in their own words, allowing them to express their feelings and opinions. Care should be taken to ensure that patients are not overtaxed or over-fatigued, and that information is provided in a style, manner, language, and at the appropriate time to prevent causing the client undue or added stress. If all these criteria are fulfilled, patients may willingly participate in student learning activities for both parties' mutual benefit.

Reflection

Learning can be enhanced through reflection, and in clinical teaching it can be the key to aid understanding of experiences (Stockhausen, 1995). The following strategy can be utilized to encourage staff and students to produce portfolios of learning supported with relevant evidence of their commitment to lifelong learning and development.

The use of learning diaries or reflective journals was strongly advocated by Nightingale to augment the learning derived from practice experience by the first students of St Thomas's School of Nursing (Rafferty, 1996). This practice still has value today, and mentors should encourage students to use it as a tool to promote reflection, and as a vehicle through which to generate questions on practice. Diaries can be essential to promoting a constructive dialogue for development. The use of reflective writing either in a diary or journal format is supported by

Jasper (1999), in that it enables nurses to develop analytical and critical abilities, and to identify their own personal and professional growth. Continual review of these diaries will enable learners to analyse, assess and direct their continuous progress throughout their varied practice experience. Fonteyn and Cahill (1998) propose the use of clinical logs as a vehicle to promote critical thinking in learners. If used on a regular basis, logs can highlight aspects of client problems and interventions utilized to address them, and through reflection on these data and rationalization of solutions used students can develop their problem-solving skills.

Judging appropriateness of learning

The appropriateness of the skill and knowledge being taught must be carefully considered. Student nurses are often enthusiastic to learn new skills that may be beyond their level of competence and not appropriate to their stage of training. It is the trained staff's responsibility to ensure that learning undertaken is consistent with legislation, professional guidelines and organizational policy. Student nurses and healthcare assistants must not work beyond their level of competence (NMC, 2002, clause 6).

Students' role and responsibilities

Students must be reminded that in the climate of 'self-directed, student-centred, adult learning' that underpins nurse education today, they are responsible and accountable for their continuous progression and achievement of stated aims and level of competence (UKCC, 1999). The use of learning contracts is again invaluable in this context in that they promote student–mentor interaction, and increase student motivation and self-assessment. By being individually tailored to each student's specific curricula, as well as personal needs, they also provide an in-depth structured framework through which student progress and level of attainment can be monitored (Chan and Chien, 2000). A continual dialogue and supportive relationship should be maintained between the student and the mentor. Learning should be provided to maximize every opportunity, and experience available. Proactive supportive measures must be put in place at the earliest opportunity, and then the outcome, pass or fail, will have been achieved in an equitable manner. The student should be advised as to the next step in the process, and be clear as to time scale for second attempts. The mentor will be able to continue to provide effective support and guidance to proceeding students, knowing that every effort has been made to help the student to achieve a positive outcome, but that the decision made was justified and fully supported.

Preparing students for the reality of placements

Opportunities should be made available for discussing expectations of practice areas with students before they begin their placements. It should made explicit exactly what they will be expected to do, especially in relation to the extent that they will be involved in 'hands-on' care. Ideal some of the nursing staff from the placement areas should be included in these discussions, but this may not be feasible due to heavy workloads. However, an alternative strategy is for a senior nurse to speak to the students as a group on their orientation day. This allows the students to ask questions and voice concerns. The principle of giving information to reduce anxiety to patients (Pudner, 1999) is also applicable to students going to a new placement, especially for the first time. Shift times and off-duty rotas must be clarified well in advance to ensure that students have time to make any special arrangements for travel or childcare. The visible presence of the link lecturer is a requisite at this time, highlighting their link to the clinical area and assisting in the orientation programme. It is part of their role to formally introduce the novice students, on their first placement, to the clinical area.

Supernumerary status and appropriate levels of participation and observation

There should be clarity with regard to both the staff's and students' understanding and expectations related to the supernumerary status of students. 'Supernumerary status means, in relation to a student, that she/he shall not as part of her/his course of preparation be employed by any person or body under a contract of service to provide nursing care' (UKCC, 2000a). Staff and students may not fully understand the concept of 'supernumerary status'. Some misconceptions prevalent may be that:

- the student is only obliged to observe practice,
- the student can choose not to participate in client care,
- it is not important that they attend for all their placement time, as they are not part of the staffing levels/numbers.

While observation alone may be appropriate in some instances, such as early in the programme, students can only gain competence by participating in hands-on care. *Placements in Focus* highlights that the students' practice experience is one of the most important facets of their educational preparation (DOH/ENB, 2001a). Clinical mentors should place great emphasis and value on the quality of that experience (DOH/ENB, 2001b). *Making a Difference* highlights the need for a 'hands-on approach' in the attainment of practical skills, which can only be achieved in clinical practice supported by trained staff (DOH, 1999). Therefore it is essential that discussion, between mentors and students, of relevant expectations relating to each placement experience in undertaken at the earliest opportunity.

Students undertaking nurse education and training courses can be likened to 'horses participating in the Grand National', as noted by McSherry and Marland (1999), some falling in the early stages of the course, others unfortunately at the last hurdle. When considered in the light of learning in practice, strategies need to be implemented to ensure that all appropriate steps and actions have been undertaken, correct guidelines have been followed and the student has been given information clear in regard to their progress and level of attainment. As we claim to be members of a 'caring profession' it is imperative that we treat students fairly and on an individual, objective basis.

Mentor's role and responsibilities

Mentors are essential for student support whilst they are learning in practice. *Preparation of Mentors and Teachers: A new framework of guidance* (DOH/ENB, 2001b), focuses on issues relating to developing clinical staff for the role of mentor, practice educator and lecturer. The principles expressed are those requiring flexibility in education provision and accreditation of previous learning, ensuring optimum use of resources. It highlights these two roles as vital to ensuring that new generations of nurses are taught by practitioners with practical, current experience of their profession. Although primarily for nursing, midwifery and health visiting, the implications will also be applicable for guidance across the range of health and social care professions (DOH/ENB, 2001b).

The major underpinning principle of this report is that all future nurse lecturer preparation will be linked within a developmental, progressive framework, beginning at the practice facilitation level (mentor preparation) and concluding with a requirement that all nurse lecturers within HEIs meet the criteria for Institute for Learning and Teaching in Higher Education (ILT) membership (DOH/ENB, 2001b). The programmes that will provide this development will be offered at postgraduate level, with mentor preparation undertaken at first-degree level. The entry requirements for these programmes are UKCC registration and completion of at least 12 months, or part-time equivalent, of practice experience.

Mentorship programme

Mentors working with students and judging their degree of clinical competence must have an in-depth knowledge of pertinent curricula issues and assessment criteria. They must also have received appropriate and up-to-date training and education for the role, with adequate time provided to enable them to carry out this function to their, and the students', satisfaction (DOH/ENB, 2001b). The quality of learning, and the assessment of competencies which demonstrate the extent of learning achieved, must be rigorous and effective.

The mentorship preparation programmes should enable the mentor to examine and reflect upon issues relating to developing effective communication and working relations, facilitation and assessment of learning, and course development. They should also provide the practitioner with the opportunity to increase their knowledge base in relation to research, effective learning environments, and the effectiveness of professional role modelling, as set out in the UKCC's advisory standards for mentors and mentorship (UKCC, 2000b).

Mentor's role

Mentorship as defined by DOH/ENB (2001b) is a role undertaken by a nurse, midwife or health visitor who facilitates learning and supervises and assesses students in the practice setting. The mentor role is outlined as:

- to facilitate student learning across pre- and post-registration programmes,
- to supervise, support and guide students in practice in institutional and non-institutional settings,
- to implement approved assessment procedures.

A mentorship model for practice

Darling (1984) recognized that the essential elements required of an effective mentor were Action, Attraction and Affect. Within these three elements the mentor should adapt certain characteristic behaviours, those of Inspirer, Role Model, Energizer and Envisioner. By adopting these and other suggested characteristics, for example Investor and Standard-prodder, the Mentor can initiate activities and actions to prompt, push or guide the learner in the most beneficial manner towards their ultimate aim/goal. This model, though dated, is still highlighted in the work of Morton-Cooper and Palmer (2000).

The mentor's repertoire of skills and experience within their practice arena should be valued for the contribution it makes to learning in practice. This is achieved by matching it with the need to know the learner's stage of progress, previous learning/experience, and assessment outcomes achieved. All avenues of support and guidance should be sought from all relevant associate personnel, for example the mentor team, senior staff members, and the link lecturer and the students personal tutor before a final decision to fail a student is taken (McSherry and Marland, 1999).

Role of the link lecturer

The link lecturer can provide clear information, support and guidance to the staff about the students' curriculum and assessment strategy. Staff in practice areas must fully understand the stated outcomes of the learner's programme. Staff turnover is often rapid in the NHS. Therefore all registered nursing staff responsible for learner development must be conversant with and understand all assessment documentation in use in their area. Comprehensive and concise written information, used in conjunction with frequent communication with the link lecturer, should keep trained staff up to date on changes, or clarify those aspects that are causing concern or confusion. The link lecturer must proactively supply this information, in the form of a pack or poster. The latter format works well as an effective visual reminder for both trained staff and learners. The link lecturer is integral to learner practice facilitation by supporting both the learner and trained staff, but in reality cannot fill the void left by the demise of the clinical teacher. This role has been reviewed in conjunction with that of the link lecturer in the DOH/ENB (2001b) review of how learning should be facilitated in practice, and will be replaced and enhanced with the inception of the practice educator role. This role will be developed along parallel lines with that undertaken by practitioners wishing to become university-based nurse lecturers.

The future

This chapter has examined some of the pertinent points related to the practice learning experience. However, nurse education takes place within a dynamic system and, as noted in the previous chapter and highlighted in *Placements in Focus*, the challenge is to expand the capacity for students to have relevant high-quality practice experiences in spite of the competing demand of increasing student numbers and the associated difficulties this brings (DOH/ENB, 2001a). Areas not normally considered as appropriate must be reviewed for their potential for a variety of types and levels of learner. High-risk, high-dependency areas, outpatient departments, drop-in centres and ambulatory care facilities are all examples of care settings that could be used in a more flexible way. Some strategies that could support this are:

- Areas can be encouraged and facilitated to broaden their availability through employing 'practice placement coordinators'. Evaluation by Hodgson (2000) has demonstrated the considerable benefits gained in improved morale, in identifying additional placements, and in maintaining and improving placement quality.
- Improved communication between key staff in HEIs and those who manage health and social care services, independent healthcare and voluntary organizations, can also expand the variety, location and extent of placement opportunities.
- The use of skills laboratories for a wider variety of 'clinical' skills for all professional disciplines could also ensure that students are prepared for the requirements of these new areas before beginning their placements (DOH/ENB, 2001a).
- Link lecturers must be proactive in 'auditing' new areas, and ensuring the availability of appropriately trained qualified staff to support student learning. They must continually monitor the current placement status for changes in experience available and where new experiences or new approaches exist, innovations in practice can be facilitated.

Having reviewed the current changes and identified the issues that providers of nurse education, both within the university and in practice settings, will need to consider, it is hoped that the learning provided within the practice arena will, in the future, be undertaken in an optimum environment. Through consideration of the strategies outlined, a review of practice will enable practitioners to ensure that it is of a standard that will enable student nurses to acquire professional competence that is both academically sound and clinically 'fit for practice', from a skills-based perspective.

References

Bahn, D (2001) Social Learning Theory: its application in the context of Nurse Education, *Nurse Education Today*, **21**, 110–17.

Brookfield, S D (1993) *Developing Critical Thinking: Challenging Adults to Explore Alternative Ways of Thinking and Acting.* Milton Keynes: Open University Press.

Boud, D and Walker, D (1993) Barriers to Reflection on Experience. In Boud, D, Cohen, R and Walker, D (eds), *Using Experience for Learning.* Buckingham: The Society for Research into Higher Education/Open University.

Bowles, N (1995) Story telling: A search for meaning with nursing practice, *Nurse Education Today*, **15**, 365–9.

Carlisle, D (1991) Take Five, *Nursing Times*, **87**(6), 40–41.

Chan Wai-chi, S and Chien, Wai-tong (2000) Implementing contract learning in a clinical context: report on a study, *Journal of Advanced Nursing*, **31**(2), 298–305.

Darling, L A W (1984) What do Nurses want in a Mentor?, *The Journal of Nursing Administration*, **84**, 42–4.

Department of Health (1996) *The Patients Charter and You.* London: DOH.

Department of Health (1999) *Making a Difference: Strengthening the Nursing, Midwifery, and Health Visiting Contribution to Health and Healthcare.* London: DOH.

Department of Health/English National Board (2001a) *Placements in Focus: Guidance for Education in Practice for Health Care Professions.* London: DOH/ENB.

Department of Health/English National Board (2001b) *Preparation of Mentors and Teachers: A new framework of guidance.* London: DOH/ENB.

Fleck, E and Fyffe, T (1997) Changing nursing practice through continuing education: a tool for evaluation, *Journal of Nursing Management*, **5**, 37–41.

Fonteyn, M E and Cahill, M (1998) The use of clinical logs to improve nursing students' metacognition: a pilot study, *Journal of Advanced Nursing*, **28**(1), 149–54.

Haddock, J (1997) Reflecting in groups: contextual and theoretical considerations within nurse education and practice. *Nurse Education Today*, **17**, 381–5.

Harding, L (1979) The Teacher in the clinical field. In Hincliff, S M (ed.), *Teaching Clinical Nursing*. London: Churchill Livingstone.

Hodgson, P (2000) *Clinical Placements in Primary and Community Care Project*. Leeds: NHS Executive.

Holloway, W (1991) *Work Psychology and Organisational Behaviour*. London: Sage Publications.

Jarvis, P (2000) *Adult and Continuing Education: Theory and Practice*. London and New York: Routledge Falmer.

Jasper, M A (1999) Nurses' perceptions of the value of written reflection, *Nurse Education Today*, **19**, 452–63.

Kramer, M (1974) *Reality Shock*. St Louis, MO: Mosby.

Lyth, M I (1988) *Containing Anxiety in Institutions – selected essays*. Vol. 1. London: Free Association Books.

Maggs, C (1996) Towards a philosophy of continuing professional education in nursing and midwifery and health visiting, *Nurse Education Today*, **16**, 98–102.

McSherry, W and Marland, G R (1999) Student discontinuations is the system failing?, *Nurse Education Today*, **19**, 578–85.

Morton-Cooper, A and Palmer, A (2000) *Mentoring, Preceptorship and Clinical Supervision: A guide to Professional Roles in Clinical Practice*, 2nd edn London: Blackwell Science.

Neary, M (1997) Project 2000 Students survival kit: a return to the practical room (skills lab) *Nurse Education Today*, **17**, 46–52.

Nicklin, P J and Kenworthy, N (2000) *Teaching and Assessing in Nursing Practice: an experiential approach*, 3rd edn. London: Ballière Tindall/Royal College of Nursing.

Nursing & Midwifery Council (NMC) (2002) *Code of Professional Conduct*. London: Nursing & Midwifery Council.

Oliver, R and Endersby, C (1994) *Teaching and Assessing Nurses: A Handbook for Preceptors*. London: Ballière Tindall.

Panno, J M (1992) A Systematic Approach for Assessing Learning Needs, *Journal of Nursing Staff Development*, Nov.–Dec., 269–73.

Pudner, R (1999) *Nursing the Surgical Patient*. London: Bailliere Tindall.

Purdy, M (1997) The Problem of Self-Assessment in Nurse Education, *Nurse Education Today*, **17**, 135–9.

Quinn, F M (2000) *Principles and Practices of Nurse Education*, 4th edn. Cheltenham: Stanley Thornes.

Rafferty, A M (1996) *The Politics of Nursing Knowledge*. London: Routledge.

Shepherd, J C (1994) Training needs analysis model for qualified nurse practitioners, *Journal of Nursing Management*, **2**, 181–5.

Smith, P and Gray, B (2001) Reassessing the concept of emotional labour in student nurse education: role of link lecturers and mentors in a time of change, *Nurse Education Today*, **21**, 230–37.

Stengelhofen, J (1993) *Teaching students in clinical settings*. London: Chapman & Hall.

Stockhausen, L (1995) Reflective practice in Clinical Teaching: the experiences of two nurse academics, *Studies in Continuing Education*, **17**(1&2), 18–28.

Sundeen, S J, Stuart, G W, Rankin, E A D and Cohen, S (1998) *Nurse–Client Interaction: Implementing 'The Nursing Process'* 6th edn. St Louis, MO: Mosby.

United Kingdom Central Council for Nursing, Midwifery and Health Visiting (1994) *The Council's Standards for Post Registration Education and Practice (the PREP Report)*. London: UKCC.

United Kingdom Central Council for Nursing, Midwifery and Health Visiting (1999) *Fitness for Practice*. The UKCC Commission for Nursing and Midwifery Education, chaired by Sir Leonard Peach. London: UKCC.

United Kingdom Central Council for Nursing, Midwifery and Health Visiting (2000a) *Standards for the Preparation of Teachers of Nursing, Midwifery and Health Visiting*. London: UKCC.

United Kingdom Central Council for Nursing, Midwifery and Health Visiting (2000b) *Amendment Rules*. London: UKCC.

3

Learning Communities: Innovation in Nurse Education

Lois Crooke, Peter Curtis and Gail Thomas

Introduction

Chapters 1 and 2 both refer in their conclusions to the need to examine innovative placement options. This chapter describes such an innovation – that of the practical application of the concept of 'organizational learning' in the context of delivering pre- and post-registration nursing education. The current political agenda provides challenges for higher education institutions providing these types of programmes; at Thames Valley University (TVU) we are trying to meet these by developing an organizational learning culture within distinct professional learning communities.

The first section of the chapter sets a contextual scene for the development, the second explores the theoretical underpinning for the approach and the last section describes the implications for learning and teaching in this new arrangement. We are aware that we are at the beginning of a large-scale change which, when successfully implemented, will have far-reaching effects. An evaluation strategy is being implemented as an integral component of the change process, to help us to learn as we go, thus ensuring we remain true to our aim to improve the learning experience of our students in both theory and practice.

The context

Political influences in nurse education

Since 1997, there have been numerous reports and directives from the government which steer the health and social care professions into news ways of working and therefore influence the educational programmes that support them. These include *Making a Difference* (DOH, 1999), which examined the way in which nurses work and the environment in which they practise. This document stressed the need for the NHS to ensure that nurses are working in a user-friendly environment, with more support available for them in their practice. The expectations are two-way, however; nurses are expected to work differently, as equal team members in the multidisciplinary team and as professionals who are prepared to change their practice in response to the needs of the patient/client group.

In the same year, the UKCC released its document *Fitness for Practice* (UKCC, 1999), in response to debates about the effectiveness of pre-registration programmes for preparing competent nurses. Before this there had been growing concern that newly qualified nurses were perceived as being unable to undertake contemporary practice unsupervised at the point of registration; expectations were that the three-year preparation programme should lead to nurses being able to practice relatively independently on qualification. This seems entirely appropriate, but a number of changes in the decade before the publication of *Fitness for Practice* had affected the confidence and competence of nurses on qualification.

The move into higher education

The move of nurse education into universities in the early 1990s had affected the pre-existing, close relationship between practice and education colleagues who were supporting student learning. Physical distances between hospitals and community areas with the higher education institutions (HEIs) presented a challenge. The perceived change of emphasis between time spent in the classroom and that in clinical areas, which appeared in the Project 2000 diploma-level nursing programmes, was felt to have interfered with students' ability to feel confident in practice (Gray and Smith 1999). In addition, the resulting separation of educators in universities away from their colleagues in clinical practice had raised questions about the credibility of teachers teaching students about nursing practice while they themselves were not engaging in contemporary practice on a regular basis.

The purchasing arrangements for nurse education had also affected the relationship between those in NHS Trusts and universities. The 'purchaser/provider split' of education from practice was brought about in response to *Working Paper 10* (DOH, 1989) and was part of the total NHS Review, instigated by the Conservative government of the day. This arrangement led to NHS Trusts setting expectations of universities which were often incompatible with the HEIs' established systems and processes, particularly in relation to the speed of change. HEIs as new partners with the NHS were often bewildered at the need to change so often and so quickly, and found it very difficult to maintain good working relationships with the educational purchasing consortium, organizations of considerable power (Meerabeau, 2001). The new 'Faculties of Nursing' were caught between wanting to respond to the demands of practitioners, to whom they were traditionally and professionally allied, and the relative refuge of HEIs, where change generally happened in a more planned, structured and deliberative way.

Changes in the NHS

Since 1999 there have been a number of other initiatives from the Department of Health (DOH) which aim to bring about very significant changes in the way the health service is managed and its integral linking with social services provision (DOH, 2000). A significant part of this is the shift of purchasing power away from health authorities to primary care, thus developing the localization of decision making (DOH, 2001). The aim of this is to put patients at the centre of service delivery by:

- providing fast and responsive services, ensuring national standards are met and that these are delivered to a consistently high standard;
- ensuring that the patients are represented at a local level and are empowered to become involved in the decision making and change the culture of their local health care provision;
- acknowledging that staff who work on the front line are best placed to understand the needs and concerns of patients and therefore know what needs to be done to make health and social care more effective;

- developing Primary Care Trusts (PCTs), which will become the cornerstone of the NHS and will work with outside organizations such as councils to ensure local health needs are met;
- commissioning by PCTs of NHS Trusts to provide care to patients in hospitals; doctors and nurses will be encouraged to form clinical networks to ensure the development and delivery of best practices across the service.

It is envisaged that this devolvement of authority and responsibility to local 'Care Teams' will lead to local decision making in the context of local communities, while ensuring that regional, national and international networks are developed to facilitate the sharing of best practices which are delivered locally.

These initiatives will be monitored by the Commision for Health Improvement (CHI) which is responsible for reviewing the quality of the clinical governance arrangements within NHS Trusts. The first round of these inspection visits has now been completed and the results published.

The government has also developed the Social Exclusion Unit, whose role it is to identify areas of deprivation and to work with the local government and other agencies to put in place measures to improve the health and living standards of people who live in these deprived areas. Again the emphasis is on identifying 'local' issues and dealing with them locally, involving local people.

This inevitably affects health and social care delivery. The Cabinet Office in January 2000 released 'A New Commitment to Neighbourhood Renewal: National Strategy Action Plan', which identified the 88 most deprived local authority (LA) districts in the country. Seventy per cent of the national black and minority ethnic population live in these LAs. This is a very different social picture to the 1970s and 1980s, which therefore requires different working practices for health, social and other agencies to bring about equality of access to resources as a contribution to social harmony, and therefore a very different preparation of future practitioners.

Many of the government initiatives have indicated very clearly that while there is a desire to put resources into areas of greatest need, this must be matched by local communities becoming involved in the decision-making processes in support of their local environment. There is therefore a need to rekindle the ideology of 'Citizenship', where commitment, authority and responsibility come together, each member of the community playing its part for the greater good of that community. It is in this changing social context that we are now preparing the nurses of the future. These nurses must be clinically competent, being equal team members in developing and delivering contemporary healthcare; they also need to be politically aware of the social context in which they live and work and become involved in the wider aspects of their local community.

TVU's context

In support of this changing climate in health and social services, at TVU we are developing 'learning communities' in which our nursing programmes will be delivered. One crucial reason we are moving in this direction is because the Faculty is a large organization interfacing within a diverse geographical area. We service NHS Trusts from the centre of London down the Thames Valley as far as Newbury in Berkshire. We relate to two NHS Regional Offices, five health authorities and in excess of twenty NHS Primary and Acute Trusts. Students gain practice experience in some 1200 placements within the patch. We recruit approximately 750 pre-registration nursing students every year and have 238 academic staff and 90 administrators on staff. Within this environment, it is difficult to maintain a sense of belonging and closeness with a particular student group, an issue which may affect recruitment at the end of their programmes.

With this background, including political, educational and philosophical drivers, in a large and complex organization, the scene is set to describe more fully our rationale for and interpretation of 'learning communities'.

Learning organizations: the foundations of learning communities

Learning organizations make 'intentional use of learning processes at individual group and system level to transform the organization, in ways that are increasingly satisfying to its stakeholders' (Dixon, 1994). This definition highlights the transformational nature of the learning organization, acknowledging, as it does, the relationship between the individual, groups and organizational systems, and alludes to the satisfaction of all stakeholders. This is a useful definition to work with, as it implies a role for policy makers and strategic managers as well as opening the way for the patient, the student, educators and clinicians to become members of the learning organization (the learning community).

Learning organizations are founded on the belief that organizations will only thrive when they have developed an ability to adapt to a continuously changing world. Revans (1982) argued that an organization's survival is dependent on its rate of learning being equal to or greater than the rate of change in its external environment. Bringing the NHS and higher education into an organizational alliance, focused on learning for change, will enable effective responses to changes in the external environments. A position is developed where, no matter which government is in power, no matter what the latest developments in healthcare or education processes, healthcare and healthcare education will remain contemporary because of the capacity of staff to learn.

A model of learning organizations

The literature related to learning organizations is extensive, but most authors agree on five characteristics of a learning organization (see, for example, Senge, 1990; Senge *et al.*, 1994, Nevis *et al.*, 1995, Argyris and Schon, 1996, Davies and Nutley, 2000).

- *Personal mastery*, where individuals develop insight into their own learning processes and refine them as a master craftsman refines his tools, enabling the individual to attain a highly developed sense of purpose and clarity of vision.
- *Mental models* involve raising to the conscious level the hidden assumptions that guide perception, thinking and action.
- *Shared vision*, building a future with enthusiasm and commitment where the future is characterized by a shared motivating image.
- *Team learning*, when individuals, working in teams, suspend assumptions and cooperate in overcoming organizational and personal defence mechanisms in the pursuit of learning.
- *Systems thinking*, where individuals cease to be introspective with a narrow vision of the world, developing rather an appreciation of the whole and the relationship between its contributing elements.

Whilst many authors and investigators discuss the meaning of learning organizations, there is a paucity of literature on how to develop such an approach. For the purpose of our discussion, the INVEST model, developed by Pearn *et al.* (1995) will be explored. Within this model, six dimensions provide a framework for the learning organization and hence our learning community:

- Inspired learners
- Nurturing culture
- Vision for the future
- Enhanced learning
- Supportive management
- Transforming structures.

Each dimension brings with it values, beliefs, behaviours and processes that demonstrate the organization's commitment to the learning individual and the individual's commitment to the learning organization.

Inspired learners   This dimension focuses around the members of the learning community having a commitment to their organization, such that they pursue personal learning and personal development within a balanced frame that promotes the development of the organization and the achievement of team and personal goals. Learning from experience in an enthusiastic pursuance of improvement, where the status quo is challenged as the norm, and where triple-loop learning is an essential feature of group and personal working, provides the members of the learning organization with an inspirational approach to self-improvement. The importance of learning to learn cannot be over-estimated.

Nurturing culture   This dimension focuses on the culture of the organization. Inspired learners want to take risks, to experiment and explore new ways of doing things, within an environment where respect, trust and open discussion are valued. Mistakes become valued as opportunities for improvement through learning. All members of the learning organization have contributions to make and their contribution is not judged according to their position in the organization; it is valued as a display of the individual's commitment to their organization and to their team.

Vision for the future   Vision statements produced by senior executives and passed down to the workforce rarely motivate. Vision within the learning organization takes on a critical role as it brings together the values of the nurturing culture, with the pursuance of inspirational learning. The emphasis is on the process of ensuring that the organization remains at the cutting edge, through the commitment and learning of its members. The vision is developed, owned and enacted by those who work with it, and provides the foundation for enhanced learning. The vision drives the quality management system.

Enhanced learning   This dimension focuses on the development of processes that enable learning: not the single-loop learning so pervasive in the current health service and higher education sector; rather the triple-loop learning that will enable the learning community to learn how to learn. Action learning, mentoring, learning contracts, learning laboratories, enquiry-focused curriculum, cognitive apprenticeships – these provide the scaffold of enhanced learning. The establishment of a learning consortium, where all the stakeholders of the learning community participate in processes of quality management and enhancement, provides a framework for learning to learn.

Supportive management   Those who currently manage in higher education and the health service are likely to have developed professionally through the Thatcher years, with its emphasis on bureaucratic, market-driven education and healthcare. The notion of the learning organization is focused on transformational leadership, with an emphasis on personal and organizational growth through learning and the focused pursuit of a common vision. This demands new skills and the growth of an open facilitative management style. In implementing learning communities, the managers become a learning set in their own right as they develop, which for many will require new skills and approaches.

Transforming structures   Self-directed teams, flat organizational structures, outcome-focused roles rather than tight job descriptions and extant reward and development systems, by way of example, provide transforming structures. Learning becomes an essential component in the roles of all those in the organization, where the contribution of the individual is not judged by their position in the organization; rather it is taken as a contribution to the dialectical process of developing creative solutions.

The underpinning principles to the INVEST model provide a foundation to the development of learning communities at TVU.

TVU's definition of learning communities

As has been described, the Faculty of Health and Human Sciences at TVU is a large organization, serving a diverse geography and population.

To date, as a means of ensuring our students have as meaningful an experience as possible in this large institution, we have placed them in training 'circuits', where they gain all their clinical experience. These circuits are the starting-points for the development of the learning communities; their strength was in providing students with a 'home' Trust in which they learned. However, the limitations were that the emphasis was in the Acute Trusts, the networks of communication and relationships were limited and did not, in the main, involve other professional groups.

Our interpretation of learning communities (LCs) has two main features: geography and philosophy. In the geographical sense, we are now reconfiguring our training circuits and developing LCs coterminous with PCT/LA boundaries in line with current government policy. The LCs will include not only the Primary, Acute, Mental Health and Learning Disability Trusts in the area but also the social services, user organizations and voluntary groups, schools, colleges, independent hospitals, nurseries, nursing homes – in fact, all organizations which can be a learning opportunity for our students. The learning communities will reflect the local community in that they will 'service' the geographical area, recognizing the particular attributes of that area and adapting their working practices accordingly.

The philosophical dimension of the LC relates to the bringing together of people in a defined community in order so that they can learn, develop and grow to the mutual benefit of all members. The university in this sense will be a catalyst for networking within each LC, helping to develop effective communication and awareness.

All our academic staff will participate in and belong to an LC; link lecturers, lecturer practitioners, professors, readers and managers have all committed themselves to involvement. The directors of nursing of the Trusts are also all signed up to the development, and nurse managers, practice development nurses, nurse consultants and practice educators will all have a role to play. A priority is to involve the other professional and user groups in the communities and to establish a forum for meeting and exploring roles.

Figure 3.1 integrates the essential features of our learning communities: the people, places and activities which will take place in each of the seven.

Outcomes from the successful implementation of LCs in five years' time will include an integration of a part of the Faculty of Health and Human Sciences at TVU in each of the LCs. They will be delivering

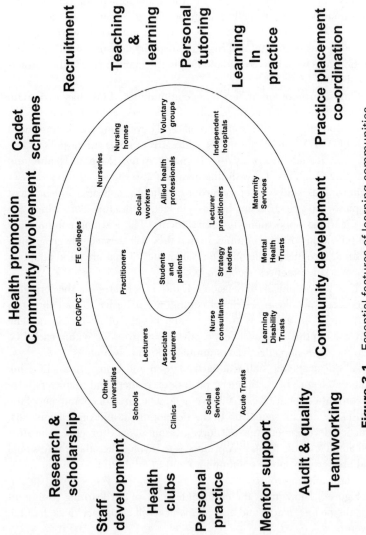

Figure 3.1 Essential features of learning communities

42

health and social care educational programmes, as well as enhancing to the capability of the community by contributing to the local economy, bringing in fresh people who settle in the area and buy or rent property, spend money in the local shops and raise their families. They will also contribute to the health improvement of the community by being a part of the health improvement campaigns and contributing to the decision-making processes in local government to shape the future of their learning community.

As part of developing a learning community there is a need to devolve authority and leadership to the communities. Prestine (1993) described those factors that were essential to the success of their communities: 'The ability to *share authority*, the ability to *facilitate the work of staff* and the ability to *participate without dominating*.' The culture needs to be open, and individuals empowered to take local responsibility for ensuring a quality student experience with a sharing of values, ideals and approaches which will benefit all members.

The evidence regarding learning communities

Whilst the evidence of success of learning communities in higher education and healthcare education is scant, the same cannot be said for school developments in the USA. Several studies report the advantages of this approach to educational change, where staff demonstrate increased commitment to the mission and goals of their employing organization (McLaughlin, 1993, Lee *et al.*, 1995), increased commitment to change and development (Bryk *et al.*, 1993), reduced isolation (Lieberman, 1995) and increased collegiate trust and joint working (Kruse and Louis, 1995).

Teamworking increases collegiate debate and discussion. A new set of values emerges, where a shared and supportive leadership enables the development of shared goals, a collective examination of the collegiate culture, and the establishment of collective learning through the sharing of personal experience (Hord, 1997). In short, the schools professional educators become a community of professional learners who, through personal empowerment, refocus their commitment from the act of teaching to the facilitation of learning. They move from teacher-centred teaching to student-centred learning. Change and development become the norm rather than the exception, change being driven by a team commitment that values and shares a vision and commitment to building a future.

The learning community model provides opportunities to HEIs and the NHS to engage challenges of the future with this avant-garde organizational approach. This approach establishes a way of working that fortifies the values of learning, competence and justice, and promotes the concepts of fitness for practice, fitness for purpose and fitness for award, as a concern for the whole healthcare team.

Learning and teaching in learning communities

One of the key purposes of the learning communities is to improve the student learning experience in practice. As discussed earlier, the documents *Making a Difference* (DOH, 1999) and *Fitness for Practice* (UKCC, 1999) set challenges for nurse educators to increase the competence of nurses at the point of registration. With the recent redevelopment of our pre-registration nursing programme, we wanted to find ways which would help to bring together the learning in the classroom and in practice, while maintaining the appropriate academic level. We believe that the concept of a learning community will help to redress the current balance to the benefit of our students.

This section will focus on specific initiatives within the learning communities to that aim: supported learning in practice, accessing best resources and enquiry-based learning.

Supported learning in practice

There is powerful evidence to indicate that very significant learning for student nurses takes place in the practice arena (Bradby, 1990; Davies, 1993; Campbell *et al.*, 1994; Reutter *et al.*, 1997; Gray and Smith, 1999). This learning is enhanced through effective mentorship by qualified and experienced nurses but, with the pressure in the workplace, mentors do not always support students' learning needs. High-quality role models from education have also been found to make an important contribution to the students' development (Kosowski, 1995; Fitzpatrick *et al.*, 1996); the role of the link teacher can be a useful tool. However, the demands put on the university lecturing staff may make spending time in practice with students low on the list of priorities.

In the development of our new pre-registration nursing curriculum, we wanted to embed learning in practice in a much more substantial way than had previously been the case. In order to supplement the teaching undertaken by mentors, we believed that it was important for students both to see their nursing lecturers regularly in the practice environment and to have the opportunity to learn from them as practice role models. In order to achieve this, we have decided that part of the 'formal scheduled teaching' will take place in practice. At this point, the majority of the programme will be taught in the university, but in each module there will be a certain number of taught sessions which will take place in practice rather than in the classroom. As an example, in a module on acute care on the adult branch, students will meet their module teacher (who will be based in the same learning community as the students) in the university. There will be a number of sessions taught in the university but, at specific points, the teacher will meet with the students in the practice area to facilitate learning.

These practice sessions will not, however, merely be classes which would have previously been offered in the university moved out into the practice arena. They will be opportunities for creative ways to meet the expected learning outcomes of the module using the real world of practice. The students on the acute care module in the adult branch may participate in a seminar where they share the case notes of a patient currently on that ward with the lecturer. The up-to-date test results can be accessed via the networked computer, the doctor responsible for the case can be invited to discuss the evidence on which the treatment choice has been based, the lecturer can help select other similar cases to discuss as a means of identifying the effect of individual circumstances on a particular disease or condition. Alternatively, the lecturer and a practising nurse could team-teach a session on the workings of a new ventilator, explaining both its mechanics of it and the significance of blood-gas estimation in the care of the ventilated patient.

The evidence on which we have drawn to be convinced of the effectiveness of this approach to learning is a 'Practice Based Education' project which was piloted at TVU from 1997 to 1999. During this project, the students on the rostered service module of the adult branch undertook the majority of their formal teaching in practice, supported by a lecturer. The evaluation from both students and practitioners was very positive (Young, 2000); the students felt that their learning was based in reality and the practitioners felt that these students were more part of the ward team as a result of their more frequent presence and participation. In addition, the lecturer derived satisfaction from the close relationship with clinical colleagues in support of student learning. Her frequent visits to the ward to facilitate the student group (extra to the expected one day per week in practice as required by the English National Board) helped significantly in the perception of an integration between both theory and practice, and university and hospital.

It was with this in mind that we wanted to embed the principles across all modules in all branches so that every student would benefit. We will continue to work on getting the balance right in respect of time spent in the classroom versus in practice, as the new programme unfolds. There are potential constraints of space and resources which must, of course, be recognized. However, the close relationships which are being built in the learning communities are helping us to overcome obstacles and to identify many possibilities.

Accessing best resources

The ENB Report *Nurse Education and Communities of Practice* (Burkitt *et al.*, 2001) identifies a series of key pointers for future pre-registration nursing education. Several of these relate to the need for good working relationships between universities and NHS Trusts, highlighting the prominence of clinical experience as a driver to both knowledge and skills acquisition. However, clinical experience on its own will not necessarily help to fulfil this expectation. Students need help to understand what they are experiencing, active support for their learning through explanation and critical reflection, and exposure to a wide range of learning opportunities. One of the priorities in establishing the learning communities is in the identification of people, places and things in practice from which students will effectively learn.

The physical distances between some universities and NHS Trusts has posed a restriction on easy access to specialists in practice as teachers for student nurses. When the School of Nursing was on the hospital site, it was reasonably easy to have a specialist nurse, therapist or doctor to come over to give a lecture to the students. With both the time-consuming distances to travel and the changes in funding arrangements, regular participation of these specialists has decreased. The regular attendance of the students in practice (in addition to their 'placement' hours) will provide opportunities for experts based in practice to participate more regularly in the teaching of student nurses without the current resource-intensive implications. Our intention is to become increasingly aware of the extent of expertise available in each practice environment through the networks created within the learning communities. Link lecturers currently have insight into many possibilities, but the collaborative nature of the learning community should significantly enhance communication and therefore access to expert resources.

In addition to specialist practitioners, students from other professional groups will be a further resource to be considered in the learning communities. There is an increasing acceptance of the value of practitioners working together in supporting patients, learning together as students. Timetables with regular scheduled learning time in practice will provide lecturers with the opportunity to pursue possibilities of linking student groups together for joint sessions where cases can be discussed and the role of each professional group in the support of the client considered.

Enquiry-based learning

Enquiry-based learning (EBL) is an overall umbrella term to describe a particular philosophical learning approach based on social constructivist theories of learning. It is based on the broad premise that deep learning, which is retained and that can be applied to new situations, is best learned when the student engages actively with knowledge, facts, concepts, evidence theory and practice. Problem-based learning, practice-based education and evidence-informed learning are all approaches which sit under the EBL umbrella. We have a great deal of experience with problem-based learning (PBL) at TVU (Thomas *et al.*, 1998; Marks *et al.*, 2000; McCourt and Thomas (2001)) from having used the approach in our existing BSc Nursing and BSc Midwifery programmes. The concepts of EBL and PBL are similar and there is significant evidence that PBL can make a positive impact on student learning. A synopsis of the strengths and weaknesses based on a review of the evidence is given in Table 3.1 (Thomas, 2001).

We believed that both our own experience and that of external research and evaluations were sufficiently impressive to want to adopt PBL/EBL as the main teaching and learning method in the new curriculum. The weaknesses in the approach relate mainly to the need for well-prepared staff and a well-structured curriculum. An extensive staff development programme has been established to provide all lecturers involved in the programme with the opportunity to develop skills in and confidence with the approach.

An important aspect of EBL is in using real-life practice as the driver to learning. The need for students to have direct access to facilitated learning opportunities in practice, in a regular and structured way, was

Table 3.1 Problem-based learning: strengths and weaknesses

Strengths of PBL	Equivocal (PBL is no better or worse)	Weaknesses/ challenges of PBL
Students enjoy the learning method, finding it stimulating and challenging	Assessment results	It takes careful planning to develop effective triggers
Many lecturers enjoy the style of interaction with students		Tutors need to learn the skills of facilitation
Students develop a variety of skills: • Ability to self-direct learning • Problem solving • Learning-to-learn • Clinical performance • Interpersonal relationships • Basing practice on evidence		Students can be anxious if the facilitation does not provide a framework
Students develop positive values: • Openness • Person-centredness • Being supportive in a group		Students do not perform as well on factual science-based examinations
Learning is retained (deep as opposed to superficial learning takes place)		

another important driver for establishing the learning communities. As discussed earlier, in the new pre-registration nursing programme, lecturing staff will be facilitating tutorials on a regular basis in the practice environment. The close networks being developed within the learning communities will provide opportunities for scenarios from practice to underpin effective student learning, with access to a variety of resources in practice to enhance this learning.

Conclusion: back to the future in a new arrangement

Despite the present drive for continuous change and development, students (and patients) require security generated by stability. They do not want to be surrounded by constant change or by individuals who suffer intolerable levels of stress, and generate the same in others, in an attempt to keep up with the pace. Students (and patients) want a stable environment and to be surrounded by facilitating individuals who will accompany them on their journey.

Learning communities provide a powerful structure, philosophy and organizational approach that enable professional teachers and practitioners to generate the stability required for effective healthcare delivery and healthcare education. This organizational approach involves a new culture, an alliance that reflects a values set focused on continuous personal and organizational learning, personal and organizational competence and social justice. Organization in this context refers to the alliance between the key players of the NHS, the local community, including social care and social services, PCTs, private healthcare, non governmental agencies, the probation and police service, higher education institutions, local schools and colleges – all coming together in a reciprocal commitment to learning. The characteristics of this new organizational alliance must reflect high transactional integration with the development of an implicit trust and shared values system. We must return to where we came from, but in a position where this future harnesses the strengths of the contemporary health service coupled to an innovative and creative higher education sector. This will be the learning community for healthcare education.

References

Argyris, C and Schon, D A (1996) *Organisational Learning II, Theory, Method and Practice*. Reading, MA: Addison Wesley.

Bradby, M (1990) Status passage into nursing: another view of the process of socialisation into nursing, *Journal of Advanced Nursing*, 15, 1220–5.

Bryk, A S, Easton, J Q, Kerbow, D, Rollow, S G and Sebring, P (1993) The State of Chicago School Reform, *Phi Delta Kappa* **76**(1), 74–8.

Burkitt, I, Husband, C, Mackenzie, J, Torn, A and Crow, R (2001) *Nurse Education and Communities of Practice*. London: ENB.

The Cabinet Office (2000) *A New Commitment to Neighbourhood Renewal*, National Strategy Action Plan. Foreword by Rt. Hon. Tony Blair MP – January 2000.

Campbell, I E, Larrivee, L, Field, P A, Day, R A and Reutter, L (1994) Learning to nurse in the clinical setting, *Journal of Advanced Nursing*, **20**, 1125–31.

Davies, E (1993) Clinical role modelling: uncovering hidden knowledge, *Journal of Advanced Nursing*, **18**, 627–36.

Davies, H and Nutley, S (2000) Developing Learning Organisations in the new NHS, *British Medical Journal*, **320**, 998–1001.

Department of Health (1989) *Education and Training: Working Paper 10*. London: HMSO.

Department of Health (1999) *Making a Difference: Strengthening the Nursing, Midwifery and Health Visiting Contribution to Health and Health Care*. London: DOH.

Department of Health (2000) *The NHS Plan: A plan for investment, a plan for reform*. London: DOH.

Department of Health (2001*) Shifting the Balance of Power within the NHS: Securing Delivery*. London: DOH.

Dixon, N (1994) *The Organisational Learning Cycle: How we can learn collectively*. Maidenhead: McGraw Hill.

Fitzpatrick, J M, While, A E and Roberts, J D (1996) Key influences on the professional socialisation and practice of students undertaking different preregistration nurse education programmes in the United Kingdom *International Journal of Nursing Studies*, **33**(5), 506–18.

Gray, M and Smith, L N (1999) The professional socialisation of diploma of higher education in nursing students (Project 2000): a longitudinal qualitative study, *Journal of Advanced Nursing*, **29**(3), 639–47.

Hord, S M (1997) *Professional learning communities: Communities of continuous enquiry and improvement*. Austin, TX: Southwest Educational Development Laboratory.

Kosowski, M M R (1995) Clinical learning experiences and professional nurse caring: a critical phenomenological study of female baccalaureate nursing students, *Journal of Nursing Education*, **34**(5), 235–42.

Kruse, S D and Louis, K S (1995) *Professionalism and community: Perspectives on reforming urban schools*. Thousand Oaks, CA: Corwin Press.

Lee, V E, Smith, J B and Croninger, R G (1995) Another look at High School Restructuring. In *Issues in Restructuring Schools*. Madison, WI: Centre on Organization and Restructuring Schools, School of Education, University of Winsconsin Madison.

Lieberman, A (1995) *The Work of Restructuring Schools: Building from the Ground up*. New York: Teachers College Press.

Marks, Maran D and Thomas B G (2000) Assessment and evaluation in problem based learning. In (eds), Glen, S and Wilkie, K *Problem-Based Learning in Nursing: A New Model for A New Context*. Basingstoke: Macmillan – now Palgrave.

McCourt, C and Thomas, B G (2001) Evaluation of a problem-based curriculum in midwifery, *Midwifery*, **17**, 323–31.

McLaughlin, M (1993) What Matters most in Teachers Workplace Context. In Warren Little J and McLaughlin, M (eds), *Teachers Work: Individuals Colleagues and Contexts*. New York: Teachers College Press.

Meerabeau, E (2001) Back to the bedpans: the debates over preregistration nursing education in England, *Journal of Advanced Nursing*, **34**(4), 427–35.

Nevis, E, DiBella, A and Gould, J (1995) Understanding Organisations as Learning Systems, *Sloan Management review*, Winter, 73–85.

Pearn, M, Roderick, C and Mulrooney, C (1995) *Learning Organizations in Practice*. London: McGraw Hill.

Prestine, NA (1993) Extending the essential schools metaphor: Principal as enabler, *Journal of School Leadership*, 3(4), 356–79.

Reutter, L, Field, P A, Campbell, I E and Day, R (1997) Socialisation into nursing: nursing students as learners, *Journal of Nursing Education*, **36**(4), 149–55.

Revans, R W (1982) *Origins and Growth of Action Learning*. Bromley: Chartwell Bratt.

Senge, P M (1990) *The Fifth Discipline: The Art & Practice of the Learning Organization*, New York: Doubleday.

Senge, P M, Ross, R, Smith, B, Roberts, C and Kleiner, A (1994) *The Fifth Discipline Fieldbook*. London: Nicholas Brealey.

Thomas, B G (2001) The possibilities of problem based learning in midwifery *The Practising Midwife*, **4**(5), 42.

Thomas, B G, Quant, V M and Cooke, P (1998) The development of a problem based curriculum in midwifery *Midwifery*, **14**, 261–5.

UKCC (1999) *Fitness for Practice*. The UKCC Commission for Nursing and Midwifery Education, chaired by Sir Leonard Peach. London: UKCC.

Young, G (2000) *Evaluation of the Practice Based Education Project*. Thames Valley London: Thames Valley University.

4

Enquiry-based Learning in Practice

Patricia Cronin and Val Dimmock

Chapter 3 discussed an innovative approach to placements and briefly introduced the use of problem-based learning (PBL). This chapter will review how enquiry-based learning (EBL) has evolved from PBL and is a method that has been adapted to fulfil the needs of a nursing curriculum in the twenty-first century. This chapter will review the elements of EBL from both a classroom and practice perspective. City University, St Bartholomew School of Nursing and Midwifery (the School) has incorporated EBL into its learning and teaching strategy in order to allow students the opportunity to explore a full and varied range of learning methods and so enhance thier experience in both the classroom and the practice setting.

Definitions

The definition of enquiry adopted by the School is 'a close examination of some matter in a quest for information' (*Universal Dictionary*, 1998). The School expands this as related to students as guiding them through enquiry and decision-making processes in order to clarify issues arising from that enquiry. A deliberate decision was taken by the School to move the focus from PBL to EBL on the basis that nurses need to examine issues in a broad sense; not all situations that nurses deal with are 'problems'. Adopting the term of EBL gave much more flexibility for students to examine specific issues related to a particular situation and consider the essence of nursing within that situation.

EBL is an educational strategy centred around discussion and learning that emanates from a situation that students are asked to address. It encourages independent learning, and gives students the opportunity to examine concepts and principles and define their own gaps in understanding across disciplines. It is a way of learning that encourages a deeper understanding of the material rather than superficial coverage. By utilizing this approach, students become proficient in analysis, hypothesis generation, and the generation of learning curves that warrant further exploration. It provokes critical enquiry, encourages independent access to a variety of learning resources, and generates group discussion. The depth and breadth of the discussion and investigation depend upon how far the student has progressed through the programme. EBL proposes a shift in the focus of education from curriculum content to curriculum outcomes. Outcomes include skills related to the development of critical thinking, collaboration, shared decision making, social epidemiological viewpoints, analysis and intervention at the macro and micro levels (Inouye and Flannelley, 1999), as well as outcomes related to specific modules or units of learning and the practice outcomes outlined by the UKCC (2000).

Each module or unit of learning should comprise learning outcomes that will be achieved through EBL. These outcomes influence the development of the 'trigger' or situation that the students will meet. A trigger is defined as 'anything that activates or sets off a series of events' (*Universal Dictionary*, 1998). The School expands this as the use of intentionally designed scenarios which enable students to embark on a journey of enquiry surrounding the issues raised. These scenarios are developed with clinical practitioners from real-life situations. It is intended that the trigger will stimulate the students' thinking processes and learning. Student groups have an allocated lecturer, who acts as a facilitator for their sessions. The facilitator assists the students' learning by encouraging them to explore issues surrounding the situation both in the classroom and in clinical practice. One or more triggers can be used or a single trigger may develop through the module or unit of learning and become increasingly complex. Although there is much in the literature regarding this approach to learning from an educational perspective, little is documented about the input that practice can have to student learning.

Process

The theoretical basis for EBL lies within Barrows's (1986) hypothetico-deductive approach to enquiry. This approach is designed to develop analytical skills through a process of logical deduction and is formalized through a framework of simulated situations. It has been likened to the approach that nurses employ with the nursing process (Andrews and Jones, 1996). EBL attempts to encourage students to integrate theory and practice experience with real situations. When students are made responsible for their own learning they are encouraged to use their existing knowledge to determine their learning needs and so further their education (Biley and Smith, 1998a). Biley and Smith (1998a, citing Happs, 1991) support this strategy and the belief that adult learning depends on the notion of androgogy as opposed to pedagogy. They outline four fundamental principles that direct adult learning:

- as a person matures, the concept of self moves from dependence to self direction;
- maturity brings an accumulating reservoir of experience that becomes an increasing resource for learning;
- as a person matures, readiness to learn is increasingly orientated toward the person's social roles;
- as a person matures, the orientation to learn becomes less subject centred and increasingly problem centred.

(Biley and Smith, 1998a, p 355)

Traditionally, nursing curricula have required the study of distinct subjects and disciplines thought necessary for professional practice. EBL allows a greater degree of subject integration. When examining a situation, students cannot consider aspects of it in isolation. This approach has become an acknowledged methodology in many medical schools worldwide (Schmidt, 1983; De Volder and De Grave, 1989; Yang and Zhang, 1991; Des Marchais *et al.*, 1992; Thomas, 1992). Nursing courses are also adopting this process (Ryan *et al.*,1992; Creedy and Hand, 1994; Rideout, 1994; Andrews and Jones, 1996; Glen and Wilkie, 2000).

EBL is an educational strategy that integrates the knowledge from many subjects and disciplines in its process. Students are encouraged to analyse situations by identifying their knowledge deficit, thereby indicating their learning needs. Through a process of progressive enquiry students begin to acquire a broad knowledge base around a particular situation (Biley and Smith, 1998a). Lecturers become facilitators of the process and are not present to deliver information but are available to guide or advise. Situations that are investigated are drawn from 'real-life' situations and are developed in collaboration with practice staff. The uniqueness of the EBL situations utilized within the School is that they are developed in a way that encourages students to find possible solutions not only from literature but also from the practice setting. Margetson (1996) highlighted that all students start from somewhere, *not* nowhere, and that student's existing knowledge is valued and respected. However, this knowledge should also be evaluated and questioned, resulting in the identification of individual learning needs.

The main underlying theory of this educational strategy is that knowledge is constructed, not given (Perkinson, 1993). Individuals construct their own way of interpreting the world and its meaning to them in order to understand their environment (Blais, 1988; Von Glaserfeld, 1989). Teacher-centred pedogogical techniques rely on the idea that learners are empty receptacles who absorb information, which is then recontextualized by repeated practice (Freire, 1972; Bodner, 1986). It could therefore be argued that if nursing education relies solely on teacher-centred pedagogical techniques then nurses are unable to critically analyse problems (Biley and Smith, 1998a). EBL encompasses the definition of student-centred learning whereby students are responsible for identifying their own learning needs and the means to achieve them. Ensuring an effective learning environment that encourages learning opportunities and the integration of practice and theory develops autonomous nurses who are fit for practice. Engel (1991) suggests that this strategy is not just a method, but a way of learning that allows students to learn a number of subjects concurrently, in context, with relevance to 'real-life' practice situations. By simulating situations that are likely to occur or indeed have occurred in the practice setting, students are able to develop the processes of critical thought and problem solving within a safe environment. This strategy dictates not what to learn but how to learn (Biley and Smith, 1998a). Barrows and Tamblyn (1980) identified six stages of the process of PBL:

- a 'problem' is introduced prior to any preparation for study;
- the 'problem' situation is presented to the students in a way similar to how it would present in reality;
- students work with the problem in a way that encourages reasoning abilities through a systematic problem solving approach to managing a real life difficulty. Applied knowledge is challenged and evaluated, appropriate to the students' level of learning;

Table 4.1   Model of enquiry-based learning

Hypothesis	Facts	Learning issues	Action plan
Brainstorming of possible causes/effects and/or resolution	Synthesis of what is already known	List of what needs to *learned* in order to address the situation	Things that need to be *done* in order to address the situation

- needed areas of learning are identified in the process and used as a guide for individualised study;
- the skills and knowledge acquired by this study are applied back to the problem, to evaluate the effectiveness of learning and to reinforce learning;
- the learning that has occurred in work with the problem and in self directed study is summarised and integrated into the student's existing knowledge and skills.

The School has adapted Barrows's (1986) model to encompass the broader approach of EBL shown in Table 4.1.

This strategy should broaden the students' ability for critical and analytical thought and problem solving by integrating theory with 'real-life situations.

Modes of facilitation

Rogers (1983) suggested that the qualities of a good facilitator include realness, accepting the student and having the ability to offer understanding. However, the role of the facilitator is also to have a shared responsibility within the group (Jaques, 2000). Respect and mutual trust between the facilitator and the students is essential. Recent publications on facilitation have examined group dynamics (Mpofu *et al.*, 1998), the role of the facilitator (Neville, 1999) and facilitator effectiveness. Much discussion has also centred on whether facilitators need to be 'content' experts. Kaufman and Holmes (1998) indicated that 'content' experts found it difficult to maintain the facilitator role; however, Neville (1999) concluded that junior students probably benefited from a more directive approach. It is possible that as students become more experienced in this learning approach they become more self-sufficient. A study by Hay and Katsikitis (2001) found that while the non-expert facilitator was rated more highly for group management skills and their students more highly in the area of oral communication, students who were taught by the expert facilitator scored higher in the end-of-course test in the topic area. Their summary reported that the findings were inconclusive, suggested that caution should be exercised and that further research was required.

Facilitation is a skill that lecturers need to develop through staff development and shadowing someone who is more experienced. This method has been adopted within the School with success. It has also allowed for those lecturers who are committed to the strategy to develop these skills and assisted those who wish to follow a more traditional path to maintain their expertise. This has been possible by implementing EBL as a learning strategy that complements other methods and allows for individual students learning styles.

The roles of both the student and facilitator need to be clearly defined and the School has developed student and facilitator handbooks outlining these. Barrows's facilitator tasks include:

- interacting at the metacognitive level;
- keeping the learning process moving in sequence;
- probe students' knowledge deeply;
- ensure all students are involved in the group process;
- educational diagnosis;
- modulate the challenge of the situation;
- managing interpersonal dynamics;
- the role changes over time – coaching/modelling.

(Barrows, 1986)

Facilitator role

Our summary of the facilitator role is as follows:

- familiarity with the situation being studied and the house guide;
- facilitation of students networking and accessing a range of resources;
- clarification of role boundaries;
- creating, earning trust (demonstrating, not over-correcting);
- active listening, awareness of body language;
- not passing judgement on individuals;

- introduction of 'novelty';
- meeting to discuss issues with individuals;
- not giving information in a didactic way;
- being friendly, creating a 'light atmosphere'.

Success of student direction depends on:

- initiation of topics for discussion;
- style and pattern of facilitator 'talk';
- use of questions;
- patterns of student/facilitator exchanges;
- silence and interruptions;
- networking and the ability to use a range of resources.

Student role

Our summary of the student role is as follows:

- application of existing knowledge and experience in order to deal with an unfamiliar situation;
- identification of what they need to know by formulating questions;
- follow-up of these questions (integrating learning);
- sharing and application of new questions.

Trigger development

The definition of a 'trigger' has been discussed above (p. 53).

There has been much debate about whether students should be given their learning outcomes alongside the trigger. We believe that the learning outcomes are fundamental to firstly the development of the trigger, and second, enabling the students to initiate some form of direction for their learning. The learning outcomes are therefore published in their EBL handbook alongside the trigger.

To develop an appropriate trigger it is essential to start with the outcomes of the module or unit of learning. Triggers are developed in collaboration with clinical staff and relate not only to the learning outcomes that the students must achieve but also to the practice experience that they are undertaking at that time. We deem this as fundamental to the model that we have developed, as triggers are developed from real-life situations and much of the investigation the students will undertake will be done in clinical practice. During the course of our initial reviews of curricula that were utilizing a PBL strategy we found that many medical curricula were adopting this approach from a theoretical perspective, but once the students entered their clinical component it stopped. Nursing has pushed the concept of encouraging students to continue their enquiry into the practice arena, and by expanding the concept from initially examining 'problems' to 'enquiry' about real-life situations, critical thinking, critical judgement and decision-making skills can be developed. By developing triggers from real life situations the students can also consider not only the solution that they deem most appropriate from their research but also what actually happened in that situation and reflect upon it. To integrate theory and practice students must be able to examine the situation from both a theoretical and a practice perspective. Having considered the variables, students find that many of their possible solutions are found in practice. Below is an example trigger, the additional information given to students and an indication of how they might use their practice experience to develop their learning.

Example trigger

Mukadis and her child, Kemal, aged four years, are brought into the Accident and Emergency Department following a road traffic accident. Mukadis has obvious head injuries and trauma to her pelvic region. She has severe deformities to her lower limbs. Kemal was strapped in a forward-facing child seat in the front seat of the car. He is conscious and crying for his mummy.

Additional information given to group 1 in week 3
During the primary survey of Mukadis, her vital signs suddenly deteriorate. Resuscitation is unsuccessful and death is pronounced 45 minutes following admission. Her husband, Mustafa, has just been brought to the department by the police.

Additional information given to group 2 in week 3
Mukadiss injuries are stabilized and she is booked for theatre. Kemal is assessed and found to have severe abdominal pain. His father, Mustafa, is en route to the hospital in a police car but is not expected to arrive within the next 30 minutes.

Worked example

Having gained the initial information in School, the students should consider the following:

- physiology of trauma;
- mechanism of injury;
- car child seats.

Information to gain in practice:

- Would the Accident and Emergency Department be informed of the patients' imminent arrival?
- Is there any preparation to be done before the patients' arrival?
- How are trauma patients received in Accident and Emergency?
- How are children cared for in Accident and Emergency?
- How are the patients' assessed?
- How would Mukadis's injuries be treated?
- How would Kemal be cared for in this situation?
- Would Kemal be taken to see his mummy?
- What other services are involved in this situation?
- What care would they have received before arrival?

Group 1 – questions to ask:

- advanced life support;
- trauma resuscitation methods;
- criteria for pronouncing death;
- bereavement theories;
- care of bereaved children.

Information to gain in practice:

- What is a primary survey?
- How is this carried out?
- Is this a cardiac resuscitation or a trauma resuscitation?
- Who would see the husband and how will he be informed of his wife's death?
- How is Kemal dealt with?

- Can the family see Mukadis after death?
- What other agencies will be involved (the mentor could arrange for the student to see the coroners' officer)?
- What happens following the death?
- What support systems are available to the family?
- What about cultural issues?

Group 2 – questions to ask:

- what are Mukadis's likely injuries;
- reason for going to theatre;
- possible physiological problem with Kemal;
- issues around Mustafa being 30 minutes away.

Information to gain in practice:

- How is Mukadis prepared for theatre?
- What if she is unable to consent?
- What assessment would be made on Kemal?
- How would Kemal be cared for?
- Is Kemal likely to require theatre?
- Can he wait for 30 minutes for his father to arrive?
- If he requires immediate surgery how is he consented?
- Are there protocols available that allows the staff to gain consent without the father being present?
- What about cultural issues?
- What is the role of the police?

Operationalization and practical issues

Background

The School has arrived at a point where there is a commitment to the introduction of EBL across a range of programmes at both pre and post-registration level. Although essentially a beginning, this is also the end of a considerable period of examining the practical and problematic issues that arise in preparing for and implementing a change in educational philosophy. Some of the issues raised are particular to our organization and, therefore, not generalizable, but many will be pertinent across a variety of contexts. The process adopted within the School has essentially been inductive and started with the introduction of PBL into one unit (module) of a four-year pre-registration degree course.

From an organizational perspective, the choice of an inductive approach was determined by a concern about the implications for the organization and its students of introducing PBL as a whole philosophy of learning, which, according to the MacMaster Institute (1989) was a precursor to its success. It was our contention that it was possible to integrate PBL with other teaching and learning strategies. Some documented evidence was just beginning to emerge at that time to support the claim (Pinto Pereira *et al.*, 1993), but it was felt that it would need to be substantiated within the context of the School. Furthermore, despite the plethora of literature about PBL, there was little practical advice on how to plan and implement the change.

The change

Using Coulson-Thomas's (1994) approach, the proposed change was defined as process improvement in that it was limited in scope to the lecturers and students in one module of one programme. Key factors identified included a higher potential risk to the students' academic welfare than is normally associated with process improvement type change, and the mindset change for those who taught it. Furthermore, there were the practical issues of changing a module, that already existed.

The nature of the trigger/case

Trigger or scenario development is a complex process of ensuring that the focus of enquiry is consistent with the curriculum and learning outcomes. Whilst the learning process itself is 'student-centred', the process of trigger development is 'teacher-centred' and relies on lecturer expertise in determining what will best stimulate the students. Furthermore, there is an issue regarding the number and complexity of triggers used in any one module. Our experience supports Andrews and Jones's (1996) finding that students dealt with clinical/patient/client-based triggers more competently that those that were more abstract, for example, policy/management/development issues. However, whether the trigger maintains the student interest for its duration remains contentious.

Thus it could be argued that even under the best conditions a prediction cannot be made about the success of the trigger/s in facilitating the students' learning. This can only be evaluated retrospectively, and even then it could be argued the judgement is subjective. Proponents of PBL/EBL would counter that neither are such predictions possible in a traditional curriculum. However, an element of trial and error is introduced which in our experience caused an anxiety-type response in the lecturers that reflected that of lecturers in Andrews and Jones's (1996) work and was noted by Margetson (1991).

Whilst in our preliminary study these risks were confined to one module, wider dissemination magnifies the issue, particularly in a modular programme. Achieving integration within and across modules is essential. It is suggested that a curriculum-mapping exercise of EBL may assist module teams in achieving integration and avoiding repetition and overlap.

Additionally, in a programme where a decision was taken to retain 'fixed resource sessions', which include large group lectures and small group seminars as well as other learning methods identified in the learning and teaching strategy of the School, the allocation of hours to 'facilitated problem-based learning sessions' is complex. The model adopted for structuring PBL sessions in the timetable was:

- Problem presentation
- Facilitated problem-based learning session
- First problem based learning report
- Theory – additional information
- Second problem-based learning report
- Preparation for case presentation
- Case presentation

Although the timetable is flexible and adaptable, there are still decisions to be made regarding the number of hours required for each of the facilitated sessions. Cooke and Donovan (1998), for example, reduce the frequency and total amount of contact time as students become more self-directed. It is argued here, however, that generalizing about self-directedness is difficult in terms of groups of students. Even among the undergraduate degree students who could be said to have well-developed self-directed skills, in that they were comfortable with information retrieval and selection as well as being able to coherently discriminate and organize their findings, there was a wide range of ability. This range was even more in evidence among the large number of students on the diploma programme and is considered a key issue for the organization when preparing for the introduction of PBL/EBL.

In adopting a model where the students' placement experience was significant in enabling them to address the problem or enquiry, questions arose as to how this would best be facilitated. Initially students were presented with their 'trigger' at the beginning of the module and, having identified areas for learning, they would pursue some of the issues during their placement. Following placement, students returned to the classroom setting to bring together or process their findings. However, the success of this approach appeared to depend on the importance students attached to addressing the issues and the length of the placement. If students were on a long placement, the learning issues assumed less importance than, for example, completing their practice-based assessment. Furthermore, students in a group were less likely to meet during their placement, and thus the focus of their enquiry assumed less significance. The longer the gap between facilitated sessions, the greater the likelihood that students would not undertake the self-directed activities key to the success of PBL/EBL (Creedy *et al.*, 1992).

Strategies to overcome these perceived difficulties in subsequent developments have included incorporation and integration of EBL into the practice-based assessment and facilitation in practice. In addition, strategies for raising awareness among practitioners are ongoing.

Lecturers

As reported by Bevis and Murray (1990), one of the most difficult aspects of introducing PBL/EBL concerns the challenge to lecturers' assumptions about teaching and learning. Even in a school which espouses student-centred learning, the change in lecturer behaviour required causes anxiety and discomfort, a reaction noted by Margetson (1991). In was in anticipation of this that the School chose a path of gradual implementation first identifying those lecturers who would support the change to PBL/EBL. As expected, lecturer reaction ranged from those who felt they could not support the strategy and did not wish to be facilitators, through to those who actively supported its wider dissemination. Gibbon (2000) noted that although it would not be desirable for all lecturers to be facilitators there was a requirement was that the innovation be supported. However, from a purely practical perspective, enough lecturers who are willing to facilitate large numbers of students must be identified.

It is considered that ongoing staff training and development is essential to maintaining impetus for change and successful implementation. Despite initial staff training, our experience reflects that of Doring *et al.* (1995), who note in their preliminary study that lecturers felt inadequately prepared for PBL.

In addition to training and development, identification of a change driver(s) is fundamental. This is particularly important in a school where PBL/EBL is one of the teaching strategies and not a whole curriculum philosophy. Queens University Canada (2000) cite the difficulties of a hybrid curriculum where lecturers are often 'too busy' with the traditional curriculum (http://meds-ss.queensu.ca)

Role of the facilitator

Biley and Smith (1998a) claim that a specific disadvantage of PBL is that the success of the programme depends on the facilitator. In our experience, issues that appear to support this contention include trusting the students and style of facilitation. In introducing and preparing lecturers, the most common responses were in relation to students 'coming up with the right answer', 'missing significant aspects' and 'being wrong'. It could be argued that such responses are grounded in the lecturers' philosophical foundations about teaching and learning (Bevis and Murray, 1990), and the perceived need to ensure that students are given the right answers. Our strategy of 'shadowing' went some way to alleviating these anxieties in lecturers, as the group process demonstrated that students were able to identify their learning needs. Lecturers were also provided with a handbook, which included 'possible' areas that students might explore. On reflection, however, it became apparent that while such a strategy might ease lecturer anxiety in the first instance, it could also have an opposite effect if students were seen not to be identifying the predetermined issues.

According to Creedy *et al.* (1992), the role of the educator is one of facilitator who aims to empower participants. However, according to Biley and Smith (1998b) and Andrews and Jones (1996), facilitation styles vary and achieving a balance between non-participation and active facilitation was difficult. In our experience, there was an implicit assumption that for experienced lecturers facilitation was a commonly used strategy in education and therefore could easily be undertaken. Yet in practice both lecturers and students found facilitation in the style of PBL/EBL difficult. Initially students tended to seek confirmation, either verbally or non-verbally, that what they were doing was correct, and lecturers stated that they sometimes found it difficult not to intervene or offer explanations. In some cases the facilitator tended to become overly prescriptive, which in effect shifted the emphasis from student-centred to teacher-centred.

Having considered the range of views in the literature about whether a facilitator should be a 'content expert', the School has chosen not to follow this model. This decision is based in part on the need to identify sufficient numbers of lecturers but, more importantly, we did not want to discourage staff who were interested in being facilitators. Moreover, the overwhelming majority of academic staff are qualified nurses and have an expected level of content expertise.

Students

The argument for introducing EBL early in a programme of study and familiarizing the students with the need to take responsibility for their own learning, and the value and functions of groups and skills of self-directedness are borne out by our experiences. Primarily, degree students who undertook PBL for the final year (five modules) of their programme became more proficient in the process and had less need of facilitator input. The diploma groups who used PBL for their final module only consistently claimed in their evaluations that its implementation was 'too late'.

Second, it was considered necessary to 'persuade' students that this process was beneficial both in terms of their own development and in respect of their future practice. Their initial reaction was one of disquiet and anxiety about being more active in and responsible for their own learning, a response also noted by Walton and Matthews (1989). Yet their cooperation was seen as central to the success of the implementation.

Initially, the first group of degree students were simply asked for their cooperation. Their agreement was in part due to the relationship of trust that already existed between them and the coordinator of the scheme. However, there was also the capacity for a change to the summative assessment of the module to accommodate the work they would be undertaking using PBL. This was considered important in terms of relieving pressure on students (Andrews and Jones, 1996). Therefore they did not perceive that they were doing extra work. Although the grades in the summative results for this group of students were higher than the previous year, no assumptions were made about the influence of PBL since it could not be demonstrated that the groups were comparable. Nevertheless, student perception of the relevance of PBL work to the summative assessment was considered important given the subsequent work undertaken with diploma students.

The PBL work in the diploma programme is based on role transition and accountability in practice, which is considered highly relevant as students move to qualified nurse status. However, the coordinator is not well known to the students and PBL is not summatively assessed, although it does involve a group presentation to peers at the end of the module. Initial response is essentially negative, with students complaining that at the end of their programme they have a multitude of other preoccupations and do not want to undertake what they perceive as additional work.

A further issue centred on students' initial perceptions about responsibility for learning. Some students tended to the idea that lecturers were reneging on their responsibility to teach, and that they, the students, were being abandoned to learn on their own. The level of this response was in part related to how 'important' students considered the learning to be undertaken using PBL/EBL to their overall success on the module.

The breadth and depth to which students addressed the issues related to the trigger varied considerably both within and across diploma and degree groups. It is difficult to establish the reasons for these variations, but it is tentatively offered that some could be attributed to the range of ability, commitment and motivation seen in all cohorts of students. For example, students in the third year of their pre-registration programmes are presented with scenarios upon which their examination questions are based. They are expected to research and prepare all aspects of the scenario with a view to answering a question on one. Students are encouraged to explore the issues surrounding the scenario with their practice placement assessor while undertaking clinical practice and identify with their assessor how this situation would be dealt with in the real world. As with the trend in PBL/EBL modules, the depth to which students explore the scenario varied and is often reflected in the grades received for the examination.

The question of depth may be a moot point given that assessment results for students may not always be attributed to the quality of teaching. It is proposed that the students' perception of responsibility for their own learning is of greater importance.

The group

Whilst it is evident that the facilitator is key to the success of the process of PBL/EBL, it is our belief that the student group and its composition is also a critical variable. In keeping with the nature of groups, our findings indicate that some groups appear to function more effectively than others. The crucial question was, how could group functioning be maximized when adopting PBL/EBL.

Students who form a small discrete group by virtue of size or possession of a common goal (e.g. degree students) are advantaged in that they have an identity and know each other. Moreover, learning styles can be more readily identified, as can group potential and cohesiveness. This in turn can enable the group to accommodate each other's strengths and enhance contribution. In our experience, however, such factors cannot be taken as given. Whilst some groups functioned well in PBL/EBL there were elements of dysfunction which proved challenging for the facilitator. 'Scapegoating' and 'wrecking' as defined by Burnard (1989) were the most destructive features seen in one group. Whilst it is acknowledged that these features had existed previously, the requirement to work as a team appeared to accentuate the problem. Overall the group was reluctant to confront the issue and ultimately the facilitator had to 'step in' to achieve what was, at best a compromise.

Reluctance to address group issues was common among the larger cohort of diploma students, where small group membership was not a constant. They were less likely to know each other than the degree students, and this tended to accentuate any group problems. Students who failed to attend or undertake their assigned work tended to be ignored or 'covered for' rather than confronted. Although in the first session these areas were addressed, subsequent non-compliance remained a largely unresolved issue. Those who did confront non-compliant group members tended to punish, for example by exclusion from the group, rather than attempt to resolve the problem. Student reflection and evaluation tended to highlight negative learning from these experiences. Comments such as 'you learn that you cannot rely on colleagues' were common.

Minimizing the potential for group dysfunction is seen as a particularly difficult aspect of PBL/EBL and there is little in the literature regarding strategies adopted by others. The question as to the best model of structuring groups remains contentious. While consistent membership throughout the programme is advantageous in terms of the potential for cohesion and group functioning, there are the disadvantages of creating a highly dysfunctional group, which may adversely affect learning.

Practice experience

There is an increased need for today's nurses to be autonomous, adaptable and flexible lifelong learners who are fit for practice and purpose. EBL aims to contribute to the development of such nurses. The practice of nursing is not seen as the end product of a theoretical programme, but as part of the learning experience (Townsend, 1990). Students practice experience forms 50 per cent of their pre-registration education, and they are encouraged to use the processes of EBL to explore the situations surrounding the patients/clients in their care. This approach encourages students to be active participators rather than passive receivers of knowledge (Creedy *et al.*, 1992), enabling them to participate constructively in patient/client care. Creedy *et al.* (1992), also indicate that students are thus provided with the opportunity to develop, apply and evaluate their own understandings of the concepts being studied ino both simulated and actual situations.

In order to achieve this, Higher Education Institutions must work in partnership with the placement providers, a concept outlined in the DOH/ENB (2001) publication *Placements in Focus*. This involves close collaboration at the grass-roots level. Lecturers and practitioners must work together in developing triggers from real-life situations which are related to the practice experience available. This requires practice staff to have a working knowledge of the curriculum and the expectations of the students. Part of the role of the practice arena is to provide the students with learning opportunities that allow them to achieve their outcomes and facilitate continued learning. The EBL process goes some way in assisting this to happen. One of the arguments used to support this strategy is the concept of contextual learning, the premise that when we learn material in the context of where and how it will be used, learning and the ability to use information is enhanced (Albanese, 2000). However, Albanese (2000) also believes that other theories provide better support, such as the information processing theory, c-operative learning theory, self-determination theory and control theory (Schmidt, 1983; Glasser, 1986; Williams *et al.*, 1999). When considering the overarching approaches of all these theories, they lead us to look again at the process employed. The process of EBL explores not *what* is being learnt but *how* it is being learnt, and this becomes an essential skill for the life-long learner. The process can be adapted to both the classroom and the practice setting, which are then viewed by the student as of equal importance. Practice staff are also motivated by their involvement and contribution to the students' learning. The example highlighted above was developed in conjunction with practice staff from a real-life situation. Staff were aware of the issues that the students would be exploring in relation to the situation and were able to facilitate appropriate learning opportunities for the students, for example e.g. a visit to a coroner's court.

Assessment

It is essential that students recognize the relationship between assessment and learning, and hence the relationship to the educational strategies that are utilized to assist in the learning processes. Assessment-driven curricula can interrupt the process of learning, as students tend to focus on what they are required to achieve at assessment rather than the process itself. Assessment therefore needs to be viewed as part of the process, not as separate from it. To make assessment more student-centred, students will need to be offered strategies that enable the development of self-assessment skills in conjunction with the knowledge of the area being studied. Assessment needs to integrate the learning process as opposed to what has actually been learned. Savin-Baden (2001) makes the following suggestions:

- **Group Presentation** – models the process but is difficult to mark;
- **Individual Presentation** – same problems and students may only present the component that they have researched rather than viewing the situation as a whole;
- **Group and Individual Presentation** – can work well and seems to promote equity;
- **Tripartite Assessment** – consists of three components, the group submits a report, the individual submits the piece of work that they have researched and the individual writes an account of the group process;
- **Case-based Individual Essay** – links well but focuses on cognitive abilities;
- **Case-based Care Plan in Practice** – effective but must be criterion referenced and therefore disliked by some staff;
- **Portfolio** – sometimes lacks the requirement to create an overall synthesis and can be difficult to mark;

- ***Triple Jump*** – individual students are presented with a situation and discuss with an oral examiner. They then locate relevant material and discuss their findings with the examiner who rates them on problem solving skills, self directed learning skills and knowledge;
- ***Self Assessment*** – students must be developed to undertake this, it allows the student to think carefully about what they know and what they need to know;
- ***Peer Assessment*** – this emphasises the co-operative nature of EBL and help guide the evaluation process;
- ***Viva Voce Examinations*** – a useful tool in practice but costly and time consuming;
- ***Reflective Journals*** – students hand in their reflective components each week and receive a mark at the end of the module or unit of learning, can be criterion referenced;
- ***Facilitator Assessment*** – this affects how the student views the facilitator and there is much debate about this;
- ***Reports*** – can promote succinct critical pieces of work if the word limit is short;
- ***Patchwork Test*** (Winter *et al.*, 1999) – encourages students to present their work in written form. They build up a text over several weeks, each component is shared with other students in the group and they are expected to use different styles e.g. commentary on a lecture, book review. This assessment has an emphasis on critique and self-questioning.

As can be seen, there is a plethora of assessment methods to choose from; however, it is important to consider the assessment method in conjunction with the curriculum.

Within the School it was decided that EBL was one learning and teaching strategy that would be adopted among many others, and therefore a variety of assessment approaches were required. As practice was deemed an essential component, allowing students to undertake the process of learning, it was viewed as appropriate for students to approach their EBL through the practice-based assessment tool. Here students are asked to reflect on how their learning outcomes were achieved, what they feel they have learnt from the experience, and how the EBL assisted in that process. They are required to provide evidence of that achievement, supported by current literature and are awarded a mark for that work. We believe that this truly helps in the integration of theory and practice. Formative assessment is also undertaken through group presentations, and students participate in this process willingly and begin to view learning as fun. Our early experience showed us that students who opted not to participate in this formative assessment regretted their decision and had feelings of 'letting their colleagues down'. They stated that what they had learnt from this was that teamwork in nursing was essential and that we all rely upon each other.

Evaluation

EBL and its implementation within nursing curricula in the United Kingdom is an expanding concept; however, limited evaluation work has been undertaken beyond that which is prescriptive and descriptive (Biley and Smith, 1998b). The benefits of this process are largely taken from the medical experience (Barrows, 1976; Feletti *et al.*, 1982; Woodward and Ferrier, 1983; Boshuizen and Claessen, 1984; Imbos *et al.*, 1984; Coles, 1985; Colby, 1986; Newble and Clark, 1986; Schmidt *et al.*, 1987; Mennin and Martinez-Burrola, 1990). Biley and Smith (1998b) highlight that it has been assumed that these benefits are easily transferable to nursing curricula. They also indicate that any evaluation of an educational technique is arduous, if not impossible: all variables must be addressed and a complete picture of the process from input to output examined. This must, by definition, include a sound evaluation of the practice influence on learning.

Here is a unique opportunity for longitudinal studies. Students undertaking these programmes with an EBL component should have their learning evaluated and the study needs to continue following qualification if we are to determine the effectiveness of this strategy, which could support not only nursing curricula but also interprofessional learning. Biley and Smith (1998b) have come close to this in a study that they undertook on graduates' own perceptions of their learning through PBL. The most interesting aspect that they discovered was the graduates' belief that their function was to become catalysts for change within the profession. They indicate that a weakness of this study is that although it has uncovered the graduates' own perceptions, it has also highlighted other tensions, such as their lack of power to instigate change. These findings support the need for longitudinal studies to be undertaken. If we intend to adopt EBL within nursing curricula, we must start providing the evidence of its effect. The only way to do this is to start evaluating the process.

References

Albanese, M (2000) Problem Based Learning: Why Curricula are Likely to Show Little Effect on Knowledge and Clinical Skills, *Medical Education*, **34**, 729–38.

Andrews, M and Jones, P R (1996) Problem Based Learning in an Undergraduate Nursing Programme: a Case Study, *Journal of Advanced Nursing*, **23**, 357–65.

Barrows, H S (1976) An Evaluation of Problem Based Learning in Small Groups Utilising a Simulated Patient, *Journal of Medical Education*, **51**(1), 52–4.

Barrows, H S (1986) A Taxonomy of Problem Based Learning Methods, Medical Education, **20**, 481–86.

Barrows, H S and Tamblyn, R M (1980) Problem Based Learning: an Approach to Medical Education, New York: Springer.

Bevis, E and Murray, J (1990) The essence of the curriculum revolution: emancipatory teaching, *Journal of Nursing Education*, **29**(7), 326–31.

Biley, F G and Smith, K L (1998a) Exploring the Potential of Problem Based Learning in Nurse Education, *Nurse Education Today*, **18**, 353–61.

Biley, F G and Smith, K L (1998b) 'The Buck Stops Here': accepting the Responsibility for Learning and Actions after Graduation from a Problem Based Learning Nursing Education Curriculum, *Journal of Advanced Nursing*, **27**, 1021–29.

Blais, D M (1988) Constructivism: a Theoretical Revolution in Teaching, *Journal of Developmental Education*, **11**(3), 2–7.

Bodner, G M (1986) Constructivism: a Theory of Knowledge, *Journal of Chemical Evaluation*, **63**(10), 873–7.

Boshuizen, H P A and Claessen, H F A (1984) The Nature of the Concepts Used in Medical Problem Solving by Students of Different Levels of Expertise. In Schmidt, H G and De Volder, M L (eds), *Tutorials in Problem Based Learning*: Assen: Van Gorcum.

Burnard, P (1989) *Teaching interpersonal skills*. London: Chapman & Hall.

Colby, K (1986) Problem Based Learning of Social Sciences and Humanities by Fourth Year Medical Students, Journal of Medical Education 14, 320–25.

Coles, C R (1985) Differences Between Conventional and Problem Based Curricula in their Students' Approaches to Studying, *Medical Education*, **19**, 308–9.

Cooke, M and Donovan, A (1998) The nature of the problem: the intentional design of problems to facilitate different levels of student learning, *Nurse Education Today*, 18, 462–9.

Coulson-Thomas, C (1994) *Business process re-engineering: myth and reality*. London: Kogan Page.

Creedy, H and Hand, B (1994) The Implementation of Problem Based Learning: Changing Pedagogy in Nurse Education, *Journal of Advanced Nursing*, **20**(4), 696–702.

Creedy, D, Horsfall, J and Hand, B (1992) Problem Based Learning in Nurse Education: an Australian View, *Journal of Advanced Nursing*, **17**, 727–33.

Department of Health/English National Board (2001) *Placements in Focus: Guidance for Education in Practice for Health Care Professions*. London: DOH/ENB.

De Volder, M and De Grave, W (1989) Approaches to Learning on a Problem Based Medical Programme: a Developmental Study, *Medical Education*, **23**, 262–64.

Des Marchais, J, Dumais, B and Pidgeon, S (1992) From Traditional to Problem Based learning: a Case Report of Complete Curriculum Reform, *Medical Education*, **26**, 190–99.

Doring, A, Bramwell-Vial, A, and Bingham, B (1995) Staff comfort/discomfort with problem-based learning. A preliminary study, Nurse Education Today, 15, 263–6.

Engel, C E (1991) Not Just a Method but a Way of Learning. In Boud, D and Feletti, G (eds), *The Challenge of Problem-Based Learning* London: Kogan Page.

Feletti, G I, Doyle, E, Petrovic, A and Sanson-Fisher, R (1982) Medical Students' Evaluation of Tutors' in a Group Learning Curriculum, *Medical Education*, 16, 319–25.

Freire, P (1972) *Pedagogy of the Oppressed*. Harmondsworth: Penguin.

Gibbon, C (2000) *Preparation for Implementing Problem-based Learning*. In Glen, S and Wilkie, K (eds), *Problem-Based Learning in Nursing: A New Model for A New Context*. Basingstoke: Macmillan – now Palgrave Macmillan.

Glasser, W (1986) *Control Theory in the Classroom* New York: Harper & Row.

Glen, S and Wilkie, K (2000) *Problem-Based Learning in Nursing: A New Model for A New Context*. Basingstoke: Macmillan – now Palgrave Macmillan.

Haps, S J (1991) Problem posing v. problem solving, *Nurse Education Today*, 11, 147–52.

Hay, P J and Katsikitis, M (2001) The 'Expert' in Problem Based and Case Based Learning: Necessary or Not?, *Medical Education*, **35**, 22–6. http://meds-ss10.meds.queensu.ca/medicine/pbl

Imbos, T, Drukker, J, Van Mameren, H and Verwijnen, M (1984) The Growth in Knowledge of Anatomy in a Problem Based Curriculum. In Schmidt, H G and De Volder, M L (eds), *Tutorials in Problem Based Learning* Assen: Van Gorcum.

Inouye, J and Flannelley, L (1999) Inquiry Based Learning as a Teaching Strategy for Critical Thinking, *Clinical Nurse Specialist*, **12**(2), 67–72.

Jaques, D (2000) *Learning in Groups*. London: Kogan Page.

Kaufman, D M and Holmes, D B (1998) The Relationship of Tutors' Content Expertise to Interventions and Perceptions in a Problem Based Learning Medical Curriculum, *Medical Education*, **32**, 255–61.

Knowles, M (1978) *The Adult Learner: Neglected Species*, 2nd edn.), Houston, TX: Gulf Publishing Co.

MacMaster Institute of Higher Education (1989) *Curriculum document, Diploma of Health Science*. Vol. 1 & 2, Ontario, Australia.

Margetson, D (1991) Why is problem-based learning a challenge? In Boud, D and Feletti, G (eds), *The Challenge of Problem-Based Learning*. London: Kogan Page.

Margetson, D (1996) Beginning with the Essentials: Why Problem Based Learning begins with Problems, *Education for Health*, **9**(1), 61–9.

Mennin, S P and Martinez-Burrola, N (1990) The Cost of Problem Based vs Traditional Medical Education, *Medical Education*, **20**(3), 195–201.

Mpofu, D J S, Das, M, Stewart, T, Dunn, E and Schmidt, H G (1998) Perceptions of Group Dynamics in a Problem Based Learning Session: a Time to Reflect on Group Issues, *Medical Teacher*, **20**(5), 421–7.

Neville, A J (1999) The Problem Based Learning Tutor: Teacher? Facilitator? Evaluator? *Medical Teacher*, **21**(4), 393–401.

Newble, D and Clark R M (1986) The Approach to Learning of Students in Traditional and Innovated Problem Based Medical School *Medical Education*, **20**, 267–73.

Perkinson, H G (1993) *Teachers Without Goals: Students Without Purposes*. New York: McGraw-Hill.

Pinto Pereira, L M, Telang, B V, Butler, K A and Joseph, S.M. (1993) Preliminary evaluations of a new curriculum – incorporation of problem-based learning (PBL) into the traditional format, *Medical Teacher*, **15**(4), 351–64.

Queens University Canada (2000) http://meds-ss.queensu.ca.

Rideout, E M (1994) Letting Go: Rationale and Strategies for Student Centred Approaches to Clinical Teaching, *Nurse Education Today* **14**, 146–51.

Rogers, C (1983) *Freedom to Learn for the '80's*, Ohio: Merrill.

Ryan, G, Little, P, Smith, G, McMillan, M and Hengstberger-Sims, C (1992) Implementing Problem Based Learning in Nursing. In Gray, G and Pratt, R (eds), *Issues in Australian Nursing*. Melbourne: Churchill Livingstone.

Savin-Baden, M (2001) *Issues to consider re: Assessment and Problem Based Learning*. Savin-Baden Associates.

Schmidt, H G (1983) Problem Based Learning: Rationale and Description, *Medical Education*, **17**, 11–16.

Schmidt, H G, Dauphnee, W D and Patel, V L (1987) Comparing the effects of Problem Based and Conventional Curricula in an International Sample, *Medical Education*, **62**(4), 305–15.

Thomas, R (1992) Teaching Medicine with Cases: Student and Teacher Opinion, *Medical Education*, **26**, 200–207.

Townsend, J (1990) Problem Based Learning, *Nursing Times*, **86**, 61–2.

United Kingdom Central Council (1999) *Fitness for Practice*. The UK Commission for Nursing and Midwifery Education, Chaired by Sir Leonard Peach. London: UKCC.

United Kingdom Central Council (2000) *Nursing Competencies*. SN/PW/PO ed/letters.n comp 1012 London: UKCC.

Universal Dictionary (1998) New York: Readers Digest Associations Inc.

Von Glaserfeld, E (1989) Cognition, Construction of Knowledge and Teaching, *Synthese*, **80**, 121–40.

Walton, H and Matthews, M (1989) Essentials of problem-based learning, *Medical Education*, **17**, 54–60.

Williams, G C, Saizow, R B and Ryan, R M (1999) The Importance of Self Determination Theory for Medical Education, *Academic Medicine* **74**(9), 992–5.

Winter, R, Buck, A and Sobiechoska, P (1999) Professional Experience and the Investigative Imagination, London: Routledge.

Woodward, C A and Ferrier, B M (1983) The Content of the Medical Curriculum at McMaster University: Graduates' Evaluation of their Preparation and Postgraduate Training, *Medical Education*, **17**, 54–60.

Yang, J and Zhang, L (1991) Feasibility of Problem Based Learning in Jivjiang Medical College: Why not try it?, *Medical Education*, **25**, 34–7.

5

Managing Relationships in Practice

Philippa Sully

Introduction

Chapter 4 has discussed the use of enquiry-based learning within nurse education programmes and within practice experiences. Due to the nature of this strategy it is inevitable that students learn to question aspects of care, and to be professional about their roles. This should be undertaken with some knowledge of how to manage relationships within the practice areas. That the practice of nursing is essentially about effective professional relationships between nurses and those they care for, their peers, colleagues in different disciplines and managers is well recognized. However, the ways in which we learn to make these relationships as practitioners is not necessarily easily explored in the day-to-day supervision of students in clinical practice.

Since each professional encounter is as unique as the people involved, it can be difficult to explore essential themes and skills that emerge through working alongside students, whether they are learning to practise either as novices or specialists. Often, relationship processes are masked by the urgency or technical complexity of clinical practice. We can unconsciously pass on attitudes to dealing with patients, clients and colleagues in a variety of contexts because of the crucial focus of ensuring the physical safety and comfort of those we care for.

This chapter aims to explore some of the skills that nurses who teach in clinical practice might find appropriate to enabling those they supervise to reflect upon and develop their capacities to make effective professional relationships.

Supervision power and practice

Rogers (1961) describes 'significant learning' as learning which changes the person. Essential to significant learning is the nature of the relationship in which learners practise.

Nurses who teach clinical practice offer students unique opportunities to mirror the therapeutic relationship between nurse and client in an atmosphere of trust, respect, acceptance, empathy and warmth (Rogers, 1961). Where students recognize that they have learning needs, feel safe enough to ask for advice, express their limitations and feel hopeful of achieving success, Rogers (1961) argues, they are more likely to succeed. Therefore, the processes which promote significant learning in supervisory relationships are 'commitment, congruence, valuing and empathy' (Mearns, 1991, pp. 117–18). These processes are also mirrored in the nurse–client relationship.

Supervisory, like therapeutic relationships, are underpinned by their focus and the nature of the power within the relationship. Hawkins and Shohet (1989) describe four types of supervisory relationships, in the first three of which the power relationship is unequal.

*   **Tutorial supervision** – students explore cases or specific aspects of their work. The supervisor's role is that of a tutor.
*   **Training supervision** – the focus of the work is education. This could readily describe the nature of the relationships students who are pursuing prescribed programmes experience from all those who oversee their development as skilled practitioners. The supervisor has 'some responsibility for the work being done with clients' (Hawkins and Shohet, 1989, pp. 44).
*   **Managerial supervision** – the manager is responsible for the maintenance of standards. This relationship is particularly clear when students are pursuing pre-registration programmes and cannot be called to account for their professional practice, whereas their supervisor may be.
*   **Consultancy supervision** – here there is an equal relationship between the practitioner and the supervisor. The focus of the work is the development of practice through reflection upon the work of the supervisee, who remains accountable for their practice. Learning alongside others and being taught how to deliver care by more experienced colleagues are integral to passing on the skills of nursing practice. Thus the management and delivery of nursing care is

scrutinized in supervision, to ensure the safety of patients and clients. This of necessity means that there is an element of assessment of the supervisee's work, regardless of whether or not the relationship between the supervisor and practitioner is one of equals. Thus the power of the supervisor is a significant element in the supervisory relationship, whether this is openly acknowledged or not. Each person in the relationship will bring to it previous experiences of being supervised. These, alongside the power in the relationship, can influence the development of new supervisory partnerships, particularly if in the past supervisors have abused their position of power. The four key elements in the supervisory relationship are therefore: 'anxiety, power, assessment and history' (Shohet and Wilmot, 1991, p. 91).

The nature and function of professional boundaries

A boundary is defined by the *Shorter Oxford Dictionary* (1975) as 'that which serves to indicate the limits of anything'.

Boundaries function both as limits and containers, and may be conscious or unconscious. They form a crucial part of all professional relationships whether or not they are explicitly stated. Some manifestations of boundaries evident in practice are: hierarchy, uniform, role, expertise, policies and protocols, contracts, confidentiality, time and space.

The parameters within which practitioners work with others are contained by boundaries. It can be argued that when these are crossed, muddled or rigid, there are implications for the effective functioning of professional relationships (Roberts, 1994).

Because boundaries are a means of setting limits they provide protection, defining the parameters of working relationships and clarifying positions. Thus practitioners are able to state who they are and what they offer. Clear boundaries are valuable in the promotion of informed choice, clarifying issues between the supervisor, student and client, the maintenance of professional standards, managing stress and providing psychological safety. They offer a means of validating and valuing those in the relationship.

When promoting learning in clinical practice, supervisors and supervisees need to be able to explain their roles, the purpose and focus of their working relationship, what they offer each other, and their aims of working together. For this to be successful, practitioners need to be able to negotiate clear contracts for working together.

The limits to the professional relationships between nurses and those in their care are explicitly recognized in what practitioners are able to offer, when, how and where. This may be in the relatively straightforward negotiating of when to help a patient, to more complex relationships between multidisciplinary team members and their relationships with the client. Where the parameters of these relationships are not clearly defined, the confusion that may arise can, through the phenomenon of parallel process, be mirrored in the delivery of care.

The making and maintaining of professional boundaries requires the skills of sound clinical practice, reflection, self-awareness and assertiveness. These will enable the practitioner to negotiate explicit working contracts with colleagues and supervisees, as well as clients and patients.

Professional relationships with colleagues

To all relationships, those involved bring their personal as well as their professional histories. These are influenced by the culture in which individuals practise, as well as the culture of their own disciplines. Cultural differences in professional practice are manifest in the use and choice of healthcare models, the language used by different disciplines and the organization of work.

The assumptions about who 'leads' the multidisciplinary or the nursing teams influence how decisions about care are made and how they are delivered. The power bases that these imply have implications for the ways in which practitioners and supervisees work together, what they feel able to challenge, change or develop, and how they might reflect upon their work.

The context in which the experienced practitioner supervises the student will directly influence – whether consciously or unconsciously – the manner in which supervision is conducted. The overt or covert power that the supervisor brings to the relationship will depend on their position in the professional hierarchy and their capacity to influence effectively the learning opportunities available to the student.

Often the supervision of students in clinical practice is informal. The student is allocated to a team for a shift, and works alongside qualified staff in the community or the ward. Supervision is provided by whoever is available at the time, not necessarily the student's named assessor for that placement. It is for this reason that students need to develop the skills of reflecting on their learning needs and negotiating learning contracts with the help of their supervisors. This will enable them to focus on the development of their practice while continuing to contribute to the delivery of care. Likewise, when practitioners take on the role of supervisor – whether formal or informal – they have a responsibility to make time on a regular basis, for the student to discuss their work with them. Making this time demonstrates empathy for the position of the student, and commitment – a valuing of their development. This mirrors the commitment of professional practitioners to those in their care. The skills of sound clinical practice, reflection, self-awareness and assertiveness identified above are therefore essential to ensuring that students are supported in practice. Supervisors need to demonstrate the ability to be assertive in negotiating contracts for working together and managing differences of opinion; they should be flexible and empathetic in allowing for reflection and challenge.

Skills for managing professional relationships which promote learning in practice

Rogers (1961) argues that for students to learn, they need 'contact with problems' which are real to them in their need to develop as competent in their field, teachers who are 'real' people rather than playing a role, and who offer 'acceptance and understanding' of the students as they are. The teacher is a facilitator of learning who provides the resources to enable the students to develop, by relying on their innate capacity to reach their full potential. This view is mirrored in adaptation models of nursing and provides a sound example of how the therapeutic relationship in nursing reflects the supervisory relationship.

Because assertiveness is founded on the belief that each person is worthy of respect, has the right to ask for what they want (even if it is not feasible) and the right to be heard, the supervisor needs to be able to address problems effectively to enable the student to make the most of learning opportunities. This is especially important when there are difficulties in the supervisory or other professional relationships that the student makes.

In order to deal effectively with difficulties when they arise, supervisors should be aware of where they are in the situation, what is significant to them and the reasons for this. Our perceptions of any given situation will be influenced by our awareness of who we are and what we bring to it, that is, our self-concept, our values and beliefs and our life-given experiences (Wright, 1992).

Case situation 1

A supervisor is concerned that, after two weeks in the placement and despite numerous requests, the student nurse she is supervising still hasn't discussed with her how he intends to achieve his learning outcomes.

The supervisor decides to address this situation with the student. In order to do so, she advises the student that she would like to talk to him during this afternoon's shift. They agree a time to meet in the ward office.

In order to discuss the situation, the supervisor needs to be clear in her own mind about the following:

- How much time they have for this meeting
- Her reasons for being concerned about the student's apparent unwillingness to discuss his ideas about how to achieve his learning outcomes
- How she feels about this
- What is significant for her in this situation. Does it have echoes of a previous similar experience of hers?
- How she intends to encourage the student to clarify his reasons for not discussing his work with her, that is, what words she will use to raise the issue with the student
- What options there are for dealing with it.

Based on the four essential components of a successful supervisory relationship described above (p. 78), the supervisor can:

- decide what she intends to say
- how she intends to say it
- when she intends to say it
- what results she wants.

It is helpful in this situation for the supervisor to:

- write down what she intends to say, identifying how she will state her concern;
- write down the questions/interventions she intends to use to encourage the student to explore his situation;
- list the options they might have to deal with the student's reluctance to discuss his intentions with her;

- identify the results she hopes to achieve from this meeting;
- rehearse how she will structure the interview and what words she will use.

Preparing in this way for the meeting will help to ensure that the supervisor demonstrates respect and empathy for the student as well as self-respect in her role as supervisor. It is important that she owns her views by using 'I' statements, for example:

> I am concerned that you have not discussed with me the experiences you think you need in order to achieve your learning outcomes while you are here.
>
> I understand that it can sometimes be difficult to identify specific learning needs.

The above situation is less likely to have arisen if the supervisor had negotiated a working contract with the student when he first came to the placement.

Contract-making skills

Proctor (1986, p. 27) argues that for supervision to be successful there needs to be 'an explicit working agreement' which makes clear that the 'central focus' is the development of the student, who agrees from the beginning to 'accept responsibility' for this regardless of the other responsibilities of the supervisor. The supervisor in turn makes very clear her or his responsibilities to their organization or profession, and both parties 'agree to develop the skills appropriate to their respective roles'.

Contracts will identify the responsibilities of all parties involved. The student has a responsibility for her or his own learning. The supervisor has a responsibility to support the student in that learning.

It is essential to recognize the context in which the supervisory relationship is negotiated. This provides support for the work of supervision and allows for another dimension of consultation and containment should difficulties arise. The pre-registration student has clear assessment guidelines from the university where s/he is a student and explicit statements about the expectations for each placement and the limits to practice. Problems can be referred to colleagues in the university.

Should a supervisor be acting as a preceptor, the context of the working relationship will be influenced by the newly qualified practitioner's

accountability for practice as well as for example unit policies and protocols about preceptorship and the nurses' contract of employment. Like a
three-legged stool, this triangular relationship between the supervisor,
the supervisee and the context or organization allows for stability in the
support of all involved in the care of clients and the development of practice.

It is therefore appropriate that supervisors have clear ideas of their
roles and responsibilities, what aspects of these they are willing to be flexible about and which they are not prepared to compromise.
Fundamental to all nursing practice must be the safety of patients and
clients. This is obviously the paramount consideration in all supervision
contracts.

Page and Wosket (1994) describe contract-making as a process of
'ground-rules, boundaries, accountability, expectations and relationship'. Contracts set the limits to working relationships. In defining these
clearly, the supervisor allows for the framework in which the student can
develop, that is, the boundaries to the relationship. Contracts therefore
need to make explicit the purpose of the relationship: when, where, how,
and for how long the parties will meet to explore the student's progress.
Contracts are a sound example of the containing nature of boundaries.

Fundamental to the establishment of clear working contracts is the
skill of negotiating. Supervisors need to address:

- The purpose of this relationship
- Its context – including issues of accountability for practice
- What its limits are – duration, confidentiality, assessment responsi-
  bilities and so on
- Which aspects of the work they are willing to compromise on
- Which aspects of it are not negotiable, such as client safety
- The expectations each participant has of the other.

Expressing these points clearly and specifically at the first supervision
meeting is essential if supervisees are to have a sense of where they are
in this relationship and what is expected of them. When negotiating the
working agreement or contract, the supervisor should set aside sufficient
time, but keep to time limits. In this way the student experiences
containment as well as the commitment of the relationship. The supervisor should clarify the purpose, limits, format, and non-negotiable
aspects of supervision, and explore and clarify the responsibilities of each
party in the relationship and how they will deal with disagreements.

Ideally, supervisors are supervised themselves. If students know this, they can experience congruence with their supervisor, who is also willing to subject their work and professional development to scrutiny.

Where supervision is focused on training, tutorial or managerial issues, the power relationship between the supervisor and student is unequal. Sensitivity to what the student might feel about this uneven relationship is crucial if the supervisor is to negotiate a creative working relationship with the student in which reflection is encouraged. Where the environment in which this relationship develops is unsympathetic to the needs of learners, it is likely to affect how the student perceives the supervisor. Thus supervisors can be regarded as critical and uncaring, whether or not this is actually the case. Students who have experienced rigid and negative attitudes in supervision are more likely to perceive the supervisor as potentially unsympathetic to their needs and anxieties (Mearns, 1991).

While negotiating the supervisory contract, both parties need to apply the skills of:

- Stating their needs clearly
- Stating what they are willing to bring to the work
- Clarifying which aspects of the work are not open to negotiation
- Addressing what they intend to do should conflict arise
- Saying 'No' with respect and empathy.

Contracts can be re-negotiated as the supervisee gains in experience and the circumstances of practice change. This allows supervision to 'evolve as a dynamic process' (Page and Wosket, 1994, p. 144), encouraging what Proctor (1986 p. 21) describes as a 'co-operative exercise in accountability'.

It is reasonable to assume that the supervisor is likely to be more experienced in these skills. Therefore, in the negotiating process the supervisor is a role model to the student – offering an example of how to clarify positions and expectations. This can also be evident in supervisors' relationships with other members of the nursing and multidisciplinary team as well as with those in their care. Thus the supervisory relationship mirrors sound working relationships with colleagues within the same and across disciplines, as well as with patients and clients.

Conflict

Managing conflict effectively in supervision can be demanding of all involved, particularly when feelings run high. The stresses of everyday practice can spill into the supervision process (Clulow, 1994). It is at these times that the working agreement can provide a container for exploring differences. By focusing on the task of supervision and the issue causing the conflict, and by being empathetic, the supervisor can mirror sound professional practice with colleagues and clients.

When dealing with conflict it is useful for supervisors to reflect on:

- its cause
- what strategies were used to deal with it, either by themselves or others
- what observations they made – of their own and others' behaviour as well as the environment in which it occurred
- what the immediate as well as the longer-term outcomes were
- how they and others behaved at the end of the interaction
- what can be learnt from the conflict.

How was the situation resolved? Did the participants agree to cooperate on a solution? What follow-up was necessary? Addressing these issues can enable the supervisee and supervisor to learn from the conflict and develop further their skills of reflection and collaboration.

Unresolved conflict can have an implicit influence on working relationships leading to hidden agendas. These can be evident group processes, such as people evading questions and feeling tense and anxious (Grasha, 1995).

Nelson-Jones (1990) describes five steps in managing conflict. Here he explores the importance of addressing the conflict, seeking understanding of each person's point of view and clarifying what exactly the problem is. This then enables the parties to collaborate in seeking solutions, and in agreeing and implementing a plan of action.

Where it doesn't seem possible to resolve the conflict, the context of the supervisory relationship can provide a source of support and clarity. Supervisee and supervisor can seek advice from colleagues in the organization, the teaching staff or the management.

Saying 'No'

In a caring profession it often feels uncaring to withhold agreement to take on yet more work or accommodate someone who is under pressure. Each practitioner will decide the limits to their capacity and willingness to help. It is not always in the best interests of the practitioner, or the person asking, to agree to a request.

In saying no, we set limits and clarify our positions. As with all assertiveness skills it is important to be direct, empathetic and respectful. It is also important to try to find a compromise that is relevant and practical.

Case situation 2

A senior staff nurse is asked by the ward manager if she would supervise a third student nurse. The ward is short of staff nurses of her grade and she feels under pressure because of her practice responsibilities. This would be an added burden. She decides she cannot take on further commitments. An assertive response would be:

STAFF NURSE:	No, I can't take on any further commitments at the moment.
WARD MANAGER:	You are always so capable, I am sure you can find a way to supervise all three students together.
STAFF NURSE:	I can see your predicament [empathy] but no, I cannot take on any more students. If another staff nurse supervises the student, I will support her or him in the role [compromise].

Here the staff nurse sets a limit but also demonstrates a willingness to help.

Giving and receiving feedback

The developing practitioner needs to learn the skills of reflection. Integral to this process is the receiving of feedback about their practice from the supervisor in a non-defensive and open way. It is important that feedback is focused on issues and behaviour, not positions or the person. In their study, Hardyman and Hickey (2001) identified constructive criticism from preceptors as particularly important to newly qualified nurses, alongside the teaching of new clinical skills. Giving feedback is integral to these processes.

Informing students that they have not met the required standard of sound professional practice is perhaps the most difficult feedback to give. However, if the supervisor focuses on the purpose of the relationship – that is, the student's development of sound professional practice, which ensures the safety and well-being of patients and clients, it can help to keep the situation in perspective. This issue would have been clarified at the beginning of the working relationship.

In order to give feedback to the student, the supervisor needs to:

* take responsibility for what they are saying;
* offer the feedback rather than be dogmatic;
* be specific;
* clarify the student's strengths as well as where they might improve their practice;
* give examples of situations and actions;
* avoid theorizsing or interpreting possible reasons for the student's actions;
* be respectful and empathetic – avoiding blaming and being judge-mental. Making an assessment of practice is different from standing in judgement;
* explore ways in which the situation can be rectified or the student can have opportunities to learn from it;
* conclude with a positive observation or example;
* consider what message the supervisor is giving about themselves in how, when and where they give the feedback.

If feedback is given in a caring and constructive way, it can help the student to be open to new learning and to take initiative in developing the skills necessary to practise effectively. Students can be encouraged in the skill of giving and receiving feedback if their supervisors promote openness in the relationship, allowing students to inform them of how they are experiencing supervision and exploring ways in which the supervision process can develop.

Giving praise and saying thank you are essential if the valuing of the supervision is to be explicit. As with giving feedback, being specific about the praiseworthy actions of the supervisee helps them to build on their strengths and have a clearer idea of their abilities. Choosing the time, place and manner in which the praise is given is important, so that the supervisee experiences this as just as valuable as any discussion about the areas of their work that need further development.

Conclusion

In promoting learning in practice, mutual respect and valuing the merit of passing on nursing skills through practice-based learning is crucial.

Assertiveness skills are essential to these processes, as well as being essential nursing skills. They underlie the development of conditions which promote learning. It can be argued that as assertiveness is founded on the belief that each person has a right to ask for what they want (even if it turns out not to be feasible) and the right to be heard, and the responsibility to treat others with respect, it is fundamental to all professional practice.

This chapter has addressed some of the issues relevant to managing professional relationships when promoting learning in clinical practice. It is based on the belief that the sound supervisory relationship mirrors the nurse–client relationship. Sundeen *et al.*, (1998, ch. 6) describe the components of this as *Valuing, Trust, Empathy, Caring or Love, Hope* and *Autonomy and Mutuality*. Supervisory relationships that offer these to supervisees will allow for the creative development of individual practitioners to the benefit of all those in their care, their colleagues as well as to the profession.

References

Clulow, C (1994) Balancing care and control. The supervisory relationship as a focus for promoting organizational health. In Obholzer, A and Roberts, V Z (eds), *The Unconscious at Work: Individual and organizational stress in the human services*. London. Routledge, ch. 19.

Grasha, A F (1995) *Practical Applications of Psychology*, 4th edn. New York: Harper Collins.

Hardyman, R and Hickey, G (2001): What do newly-qualified nurses expect from preceptorship? Exploring the perspective of the preceptee, *Nurse Education Today*, **21**, 58–64.

Hawkins, P and Shohet, R (1989) *Supervision in the Helping Professions*. Milton Keynes: OU Press.

Mearns, D (1991) On Being a Supervisor. In Dryden, W and Thorne, B (eds), *Training and Supervision for Counselling in Action*. London: Sage, ch. 8.

Nelson-Jones, R (1990) *Human Relationship Skills*, 2nd edn. London. Cassell.

Page, S and Wosket, V (1994) *Supervising the Counsellor. A Cyclical Model*. London: Routledge.

Proctor, B (1986): Supervision: A Co-operative Exercise in Accountability. In Marken, M and Payne, M (eds), *Enabling and Ensuring: Supervision in Practice*. Leicester: National Youth Bureau.

Roberts, Z V (1994) The organization of work: contributions from open systems theory. In Obholzer, A and Roberts, V Z (eds.) *The Unconscious at Work: Individual and organizational stress in the human services*. London. Routledge, ch. 4.

Rogers, C (1961) *On Becoming a Person*. London: Constable.

Shohet, R and Wilmot, J (1991) The Key Issue in the Supervision of Counsellors: The Supervisory Relationship. In Dryden, W and Thorne, B (eds) *Training and Supervision for Counselling in Action*. London: Sage, ch. 6.

Shorter Oxford Dictionary (1975). Oxford. Oxford University Press.

Sundeen, S J, Stuart, G W, Rankin, E A D and Cohen, S A (1998) Nurse-Client Interaction: Implementing 'The Nursing Process', 6th edn. St Louis: Mosby, ch. 6.

Wright, B (1992) Skills for Caring: Communication Skills. Edinburgh: Churchill Livingstone, ch. 2.

6

Assessment of Learning in Practice

Pam Parker

Introduction

The previous chapters have discussed a range of activities to support learning in practice and some of the issues associated with the different relationships that support these activities. This chapter will bring some of these issues together by focusing on the assessment of learning in practice.

The assessment of practice has been the subject of debate in the literature and among practitioners for many years (Wood, 1982; Benner, 1984; Andrusyszyn 1989; Boud, 1990; Coates and Chambers, 1992; Fox-Young, 1995, Chambers, 1998). Issues have been raised about a variety of aspects of assessing practice, ranging from the reasons practice is assessed and what is being assessed, to the tools and activities used to assess practice, to who should assess it. This chapter will not debate these issues further but will provide an overview of these areas and some practical advice for undertaking the assessment of learning in practice.

What is being assessed in practice?

The literature about assessment of any learning highlights the multiple purposes this serves (Rowntree, 1987; Atkins *et al.*, 1993). Atkins *et al.* (1993) and Rowntree (1987) discuss the reasons for assessment as including motivating students, diagnosing strengths and weaknesses, establishing progress and providing feedback, establishing the level of achievement, predicting a student's likely performance and maintaining standards.

The need to assess learning in practice specifically for nursing, midwifery and health visiting is related to the fact that these are practice-based professions. In pre-registration programmes this is supported with regulations that state that in order to enter any part of the UKCC Register the student must have completed a minimum number of hours in practice as well as theory. The practitioners who register with the NMC need to be able to fulfil the clauses of the NMC *Code of Professional Conduct* (2002), which includes providing safe care which is not detrimental to the patients/clients and which ensures that a minimum level of performance is demonstrated.

Although the *Code of Professional Conduct* (NMC, 2002) and the Nurses, Midwives and Health Visitors Act (1983) specify some of the outcomes and competencies these practitioners should have, there has been a lack of clarity related to exactly what skills should be assessed. Because of increasing concerns in this area, the English National Board for Nursing, Midwifery and Health Visiting (ENB) commissioned a research study to examine some of the issues; this was published in 1993 as the Ace report. The *Ace Report* (Bedford *et al.*, 1993) discussed the lack of clarity surrounding the assessment of practice, and one of its recommendations was that certain skills should be assessed in practice for all programmes. These skills are outlined in Figure 6.1.

Despite the *Ace Report* (1993) and the guidance available to all institutions where pre-registration education is provided, there were still concerns about the parity and standards of the outcomes across the

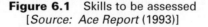

Practical/technical skills
Communication skills
Interpersonal skills
Organizational skills
Safe practice
Knowledge base
Critical thinking skills
Function as a member of a team
Professional attitude
Motivation
Enthusiasm
Confidence

Figure 6.1   Skills to be assessed
[*Source: Ace Report* (1993)]

range of programmes of education. In addition, concerns were voiced about students qualifying with limited competence in a range of clinical skills, and so the UKCC commissioned a review of pre-registration education. The review was undertaken and its recommendations were published in the report *Fitness for Practice* (UKCC, 1999). Among the recommendations was one suggesting that there was a need for an outcomes-based competency approach to the assessment of practice. Following the publication of *Fitness for Practice*, the UKCC published outcomes for entry to the branch programmes that all students had to achieve and competencies for entry to the UKCC Register. These outcomes and competencies were grouped into four domains: professional/ethical practice; care delivery; care management; and personal/professional development. On close examination the outcomes, competencies and domains encompass the skills outlined by the earlier Ace Report (1993), but emphasize these areas and provide a clear set of criteria for these programmes to assess.

This move to competency-based assessment gave clearer guidance nationally on the competencies that all students should achieve by registration, but also emphasized the need to ensure that these new practitioners could demonstrate competence in a range of clinical skills. This led to the introduction of skills schedules within many programmes that will enable students to demonstrate such skills.

In continuing professional development programmes there was some lack of clarity surrounding the outcomes on completion of the programme. Many programmes require practitioners to be able to demonstrate competence at certain clinical skills, but the programmes do not specify a minimum number of hours' practice that should be achieved in order to do this. This was solved in part when the national boards for nursing, midwifery and health visiting reviewed the framework for post-registration education. In 1990 the ENB published the new requirements for post-registration education, which became known as the Higher Award. Within the guidelines for the framework were ten key characteristics which practitioners were to achieve in the Higher Award, and learning outcomes for each were identified. Although as time has progressed schools of nursing and midwifery still use this guidance, there is the additional work from the Quality Assurance Agency which focuses on academic levels of education and expectations of students. The learning outcomes from the QAA (2001) give further guidance related to the expectations of a graduate at each level.

Another issue related to what is being assessed that has generated much debate in the literature is that of competence (Messick, 1984; Newble, 1992; Bedford *et al.*, 1993; While, 1994; Bradshaw, 1997; Girot, 2000). Often, when assessment of practice is discussed, competence is mentioned in terms of the level of achievement. In the *Ace Report* (1993) there is a discussion about the difficulties of assessing competence in part due to the confusion about a clear definition and meaning of competence as opposed to performance. Messick (1984) and Newble (1992) discuss these two terms and clarify the meaning of competence as what a person knows or should be able to do under ideal circumstances, therefore their potential or capacity, whereas performance is about the nature and quality of actual behaviour, what a person actually does in a real-life context. It is suggested in the literature that both should be assessed (Bedford *et al.*, 1993, While, 1994; Bradshaw, 1997).

Lastly, the actual assessment in terms of whether the student is assessed on a 'one-off' performance or over a prolonged period of time has been debated (Quinn, 2000; Neary, 2001). Before 1971 the General Nursing Council (GNC) appointed examiners to undertake assessment of practice in classrooms under examination conditions. This was criticized for being unrealistic and removed from practice. In an attempt to solve these issues, the assessments were taken back to the practice placements but were undertaken as 'one-off' performances, usually assessed by a lecturer or senior nurse rather than someone from that practice. Again these assessments were criticized for remaining unrealistic and staged rather than based upon someone's continued performance. This led the way to the introduction of continuous clinical assessment, which still exists today, although often complemented by other assessments. Continuous clinical assessment is based in the practice area, so takes account of the context of that practice, is assessed by the practitioners who work in the areas and who have an awareness of the issues that could affect practice, and assesses someone's everyday performance rather than a rehearsed 'one- off' example. Even this approach is criticized for being 'discontinuous' in nature because the assessor finds it difficult to spend sufficient time with the student to make the assessment anything other than a 'snapshot' of their skills, and for introducing aspects of subjectivity (Nicklin and Kenworthy, 2000). However, there is one aspect of continuous assessment that is particularly important: students are encouraged to self-assess their performance and to make judgements about their needs and their achievements (Chambers, 1998).

Tools to assess learning in practice

The previous section has identified what is being assessed and has argued that this should be done through continuous assessment. The tools to facilitate this need exploring. The literature is abundant with discussions of different tools, which include models and frameworks that enable students to be graded against predetermined criteria and their progression to be seen (Bondy, 1983; Benner, 1984; While, 1994), simulations through objective structured clinical examination (OSCE) (While, 1994; Nicol and Freeth, 1998; Priest and Roberts, 1998;), learning contracts (Toohey *et al.*, 1996; Priest and Roberts, 1998) and portfolios (Glen and Hight, 1992, Gerrish, 1993; Jasper, 1995). Each of these tools can be used to assessg practice, but the information gained from each may differ, as may the person who assesses the information.

In terms of the tools outlined, OSCEs move the context of the assessment back to the previous situation – away from the traditional practice area and into a simulated environment. However, OSCEs are now becoming increasingly fashionable within assessment strategies for a range of programmes. OSCEs were introduced for a range of reasons, but mainly in response to concerns about the range of practice experiences students undertook and therefore the range of assessors involved in the assessment of practice and the subjectivity and reliability of practice-based assessment. This tool is seen as providing acceptable levels of objectivity, reliability and validity in comparison with other methods, in part because the assessors are nursing and midwifery lecturers (Nicol and Freeth, 1998). The OSCE can therefore be a useful tool to complement the practice assessments in clinical areas, but may be inadequate as a sole method because it does not accurately replicate the ward environment (Priest and Roberts, 1998).

The remaining tools outlined place the context of the assessment within the practice environment although some aspects of the assessment may be assessed away from practice, such as reflective work, which may be assessed by a lecturer. The models and frameworks used most commonly are used in conjunction with outcomes or objectives. One example of this is Benner's (1984) framework, in which practitioners develop incrementally through five stages from novice to expert, linked to the experiences the practitioner is exposed to and the learning that is gained from this. For each stage there is an indication of the practitioner's ability in terms of skill and knowledge, as well as the supervision the practitioner needs. The assessor, who tends to be the practitioner, can use the tool to identify a student's achievement of their outcomes against predetermined criteria.

Such an approach can be seen to be objective in terms of predetermined criteria, so that the student's performance is measured against these, but one of the major criticisms of this tool is the subjective element, which enters this assessment when different assessors then undertake this 'measurement' in the light of their own experience and views. This is not a problem on an individual basis as much as it is when used across a multitude of practice areas by a range of assessors. Another problem with these types of tools is that the measurement can only be as accurate as the outcomes selected for measurement; Benner (1984) identified this when discussing her own model. On a positive note, one of the strengths of these tools is that they are developed specifically taking into account the context within which clinical care is given (Benner, 1984; English, 1993).

Learning contracts are another tool that have been used increasingly to support practice-based assessments. Students use these to outline how they will achieve the outcomes set for placements. They enable the student and assessor to discuss what the student will do in terms of actions and the evidence will then be used to demonstrate achievement of the outcomes. Learning contracts are useful for integrating theory and practice, allowing flexibility of student choice and engendering high commitment and motivation (Toohey *et al.*, 1996).

Portfolios are the last tool that will be discussed, and these link well with the use of learning contracts and reflective practice. The aim of a portfolio is to maximize learning by enabling students to continually monitor and review their progress. Students can identify their own learning needs in relation to particular aspects of their programme, such as practice placements, the resources and actions to achieve these needs, the integration of theory with practice experience and the use of the documented reflections for dialogue with their peers, practitioners and educators (Glen and Hight, 1992; Gerrish, 1993; Jasper, 1995).

Activities in practice that can be used to assess learning

The majority of the tools outlined rely upon the assessment being undertaken in the placement area with the assessors being the practitioners who work in the placements. The use of a model, learning contract or portfolio is dependent upon the student having some outcomes to be assessed, and undertaking a range of activities to achieve those outcomes. It is these activities that will now be discussed.

Rowntree (1987) discussed assessment as being undertaken whenever one person is in some kind of interaction, direct or indirect, with another who is conscious of obtaining and interpreting information about the knowledge and understanding or abilities and attitudes of the first person. There are three main sources for this information: observation; verbal and non-verbal interaction, and written evidence. These three sources will be outlined in terms of activities that will provide this information and the value of the information.

People usually think that assessing students involves observing their practice in relation to practical caring skills, and this is the most common activity. It can be undertaken both while working with the student and from a distance. It can, however, be used with other activities, such as observing the student's relationship and interpersonal skills with the patients/clients, their relatives, other members of the nursing/midwifery team and other healthcare professionals. This is vital in ensuring that the student can provide care but also that they can develop a relationship with those who are involved in that care. Observation is central to assessing a student's learning in practice, but there are many other activities that can contribute to the overall assessment of learning. Many of these activities occur as part of everyday life in the practice setting.

Direct interaction with the student through discussion, questioning and the hand over of the care of a patient from student to assessor enables another type of information to be gained that contributes to the assessment process. Through discussing the care the student provides and asking questions, the assessor can gain insight into the student's understanding of that care and the rationale supporting it. The assessor can also identify any gaps in the student's knowledge and discuss how the student was intending to gain this knowledge. The hand over of the care they have provided also enables this information to be gained, but in addition enables their interaction with their peers and the quality of the information they give to be assessed. Initially some of these activities may be on an individual basis between the student and the assessor, but as the student becomes more senior this may progress to other members of the team, the shift handover and teaching of junior students.

Written evidence is the last source of information identified. Students contribute to a range of written documents, from assessment documentation to observation charts to reports on a patient's care during a shift. The assessor can gain insight from these documents into the student's accuracy and detail in recording care and observations, as well as into the care the student has provided. These documents also indicate which aspects of care the student feels are important in terms of documenting the care and ensuring that it is available to other members of the team.

All these sources need to be used if any assessment of learning in practice is to truly capture the whole experience and be continuous. The activities discussed and the tools used for assessment of practice, except the OSCE, have very clear implications for both the assessor and the student in terms of responsibility; these will be discussed in the next section.

Mentor/assessor and student responsibility in assessment

The move towards continuous assessment in the 1970s and 1980s has many implications for clinical staff, which continue to increase with each rise in student numbers. The assessment of practice became the responsibility of the clinical staff rather than lecturers, which placed great importance upon their judgement of a student's suitability to practise. Courses were developed to assist in the preparation of staff for these roles, which became standardized as the ENB 997/998 teaching and assessing in clinical practice course, and no practitioner who has not undertaken one of these courses or any equivalent course can be an assessor for a student's practice-based assessment.

Neary (1999) found when asking future assessors during their preparation about their needs that the area they most wanted more information about was continuous assessment and how to do their job effectively. However, the ENB 997/998 course has not always been seen as preparing staff adequately for their role as assessors particularly in terms of the assessment process. In the ENB 997/998 courses the focus has been on both teaching and assessing where skills are less student-centred and supportive. There was a clear distinction between the role of mentor to guide learning and assessor to assess the student's progress. The new guidance for mentor and teacher preparation published by the Department of Health and ENB (2001) has shifted the focus to a more student-centred emphasis, with the facilitation, support and assessment of learning seen as integral to the student's placement experience. The new guidelines now refer to a mentor only, who will undertake the guidance, support and assessment of the student.

Principles and process

With the emphasis upon the practice mentor, this section discusses this role and the principles and processes that this person needs to adhere to.

The overriding principle in terms of the assessment of practice is that the mentor undertakes the assessment of a student objectively and within the regulations and guidance of the system in use. The mentor needs to have a good knowledge of whatever tool is used within the programme(s) students are undertaking. The process of the assessment interaction throughout student's placement should contain the following stages:

- First meeting – setting the scene, discussing opportunities and needs, identifying the outcomes that are to be achieved and agreeing regular review of progress meetings
- Review meetings – at least an intermediate one, where progress with the outcomes and any issues about performance are discussed
- Final meeting – discussion of progress and achievement of outcomes and any final aspects for future development.

This process is an effective method for developing the student's self-assessment skills with the emphasis upon them identifying their needs and their progress. All these stages, meetings and the progress of the student must be documented. Each of these stages will be discussed in more detail with the documentation for each stage outlined.

First meeting

When the student first arrives on the placement, the mentor and student need an opportunity to spend some time together as early as possible so that the expectations of both can be outlined and the opportunities and needs identified. This should happen ideally within the first week of the placement. The student and mentor need to discuss the placement, the opportunities that are available for learning in this placement and the student's outcomes, so that their compatibility with the opportunities are outlined. The meeting should also include some discussion of their respective roles and expectations. This includes ensuring that the student recognizes the importance of having their assessment documentation available for all meetings where progress will be reviewed.

Future plans for working together and meetings to review progress should be identified at this stage rather than be left to chance. Practice area workloads are unpredictable and so arrangements may be changed, but it is stressful for all concerned if no arrangements are made and time goes by until it is the student's last week in placement and no review has taken place. In addition the mentor should discuss the team's centrality to the care of the patients/clients, pointing out that the student may work with other members of the team, who will be asked about the student's progress as part of the progress review and for the final assessment.

The details of the first meeting should be recorded in the student's documentation for assessment, along with any plans that have been agreed. This enables the student to go away and reflect upon the opportunities available and consider how the outcomes can be achieved using these opportunities. It also enables the mentor to clear references when reviewing the student's progress at later meetings.

Review meetings

Review meetings should be undertaken at appropriate times in relation to the student's placement experience. If a student is only in the placement for four to six weeks, then there may only be time to meet once for a review in the middle of this time. For longer placements mentors and students should arrange to meet every three to four weeks to ensure that any issues can be fully addressed. If there are concerns, ideally these should be addressed as soon as possible, so that both the student and mentor can discuss it and develop plans to solve any potential problems.

The review meetings should consider the student's outcomes and their progress towards achieving them. The mentor should highlight any aspects where further work is needed or where there are positive developments. The student can discuss any difficulties they have had with trying to achieve their outcomes and any areas they feel they have developed. These meetings provide a forum for discussing issues if a student is failing to achieve and needs to have further development of aspects of their practice identified (student failure will be discussed in further detail later in this chapter). Plans for the next few weeks or earlier if there is an issue of safety should be reviewed, redeveloped or agreed. Again, all this needs to be documented clearly, so that both the mentor and student are clear about the plans. This is essential if there are problems in terms of student achievement and a possible failure of the outcomes for the placement.

Final meeting

The final meeting is the most important in terms of the student's assessment. It should be arranged for the last week of the placement but preferably at the beginning of the week to take into account unforeseen circumstances, such as sickness. The meeting should encompass several aspects of the assessment process. The student should be asked to discuss their progress and how they feel in terms of achieving their outcomes, perhaps discussing some examples from the placement experience or some forms of documentary evidence. The student may also be asked about their achievement in terms of the model if one is used and the level at which they feel they have achieved.

The assessor should then provide feedback for the student, including any feedback from the other members of the team. The assessor may again use examples from practice and documentation to support the discussion. The assessor should then give their view of the student's performance and discuss the final decision in relation to the passing or failing of the assessment, giving reasons. All this should be written in the student's assessment documents (written feedback for assessment documentation will be dealt with in more detail later in this chapter).

The final meeting is also an appropriate forum for the student to give the mentor any feedback in relation to the experience, the opportunities offered and the support available. This is often done after a student leaves a placement and via an evaluation form that the practice staff may never see. However, if the right relationship is developed between the assessor and the mentor at the beginning, the student will probably feel able to provide this feedback personally.

Written documentation

The verbal discussions between mentor and student are essential to the assessment process; however, written feedback on the assessment documentation is required demonstrate that the student has achieved their outcomes for a placement. It is this evidence which is scrutinized in order to process a student through an examination board as a pass or fail.

The documentation should demonstrate that all the above processes of first meeting, review meeting(s) and final meeting have taken place. There should be evidence of the plans discussed, any issues that have arisen and the final assessment of achievement of outcomes. It is usual for all students, irrespective of the assessment tool used, to have some form of written report on completion of their placements. This report is very important in terms of the student's achievement, both for their future development but also for lecturers who may be writing references using past placement reports to indicate what practice placement skills students have gained or if they have a particular strength. However, these reports are often written in very general terms, such as '*works well within the team'* and *'has good communication skills'*, which, once the student has left the placement, may not always mean very much, particularly without any examples of these comments.

The report should indicate clearly any areas that the student has particular strengths with an example, such as *'communicates well with patients and relatives, providing clear and detailed instructions about care and treatment'*.

Areas where further development may be needed should also be indicated, again with examples, such as *'provides a high standard of care but needs to pay more attention to specific details, such as ensuring all have their drinks etc. left near them once care is completed'*. Lastly, an overall comment about the student is useful, such as that the student is at the level expected for their stage of the programme.

Providing detailed, clear and specific feedback is time-consuming for a mentor but shows their interest in that student, gives them clear feedback on their performance in the placement and their achievements, but also enables them to use it for their future development. In addition, if a student has had difficulties, it shows the actions the mentor took to support them, and if they fail, it indicates all the plans agreed to enable them to develop their practice to a level at which they could pass. This is particularly important if a student makes an appeal.

Failing a student

Students generally enjoy their placement experiences and very rarely does a student fail a practice-based assessment, which is why when it happens it is a stressful experience for all involved. The programme and stage of that programme do not make a difference when it comes to student failure: it is equally difficult whether the student is a first placement student or a post-registration course student. All sorts of feeling are associated with the failure of an assessment for both for the mentor and the student. For the mentor such feelings are usually associated with guilt in relation to whether enough support was offered or whether problems were identified early enough. If the principles and processes outlined above have been followed, then the final decision to fail the student will be fair and objective. Outlined here will be the additional steps that need to be integrated into the above process if the student is going to fail their practice-based assessment.

The first meeting should take place as discussed and the plans documented as outlined. It may well be early into the placement that a problem first occurs, and the first review meeting should then be called even if it has been agreed previously that this will happen later. This is so that the mentor can raise the issues early and enable the student to respond to them as well as review the plans that have been made for the student so that they include this issue. Whatever the issue is, examples should be given to the student and included in any documentation. Students must be given the opportunity as early as possible to correct any aspects of their performance that have raised concern. It is also essential that, having identified the problem and agreed plans to resolve it, another meeting is set up to review the progress with this plan within a week. At this stage this is sufficient action, unless the problem has not been identified until very late in the student's placement experience. If this is the case, then liaison with an appropriate member of the school/university staff should occur at this point.

At the review meeting the plans should be discussed and the student's progress to this point. If the issue has been resolved, then this can be documented and no further plans are needed. However, if there appears to be no improvement, further action is necessary. This action may consist of several steps. First, the student and mentor need to agree a new plan of action and document this clearly with a statement that the issue is unresolved. Second, the appropriate person from the school/university should be contacted. This person may vary in institutions, from the student's personal tutor to a link lecturer to a lecturer responsible for practice. The role of this person is not as important as the action of informing them. This person can provide support for the mentor and may come and see the student to discuss the issue, or come and work with the student. The essential point is that someone has been informed of the problem and is aware that a student may be failing their practice-based assessment. This enables the correct action to be taken at the final meeting.

There may be just the one review meeting before the final meeting or there may be several, depending upon the length of placement the student in undertaking. This is not an issue, except that if a problem does not occur until well into the placement, the student and mentor have less time to develop this area.

At the final meeting the decision is made about the student's performance, and in particular the aspect of their performance that has raised concerns. The issue may have been resolved, which will be documented, and then the student may receive a pass. However, it may not have been resolved, and the student may fail their practice-based assessment. If the final decision is failure, then the student must be very clear about what they have failed and why. The mentor should give examples of the issues and discuss why the failure has been given. The discussion should also include some advice about correcting the problem in a future assessment. All of this should be carefully documented and signed by both the student and mentor. The person who has already had some involvement from the school/university should also be notified of the final decision.

Students usually have two opportunities to undertake assessments, so if this is their first failure they will be given a chance to resubmit the assessment following further development, which may be in the same placement or another, depending on the policy of the institution. However, if this is the student's second attempt, they may well be discontinued, which is appropriate if a student has failed twice despite advice, support and clear action and documentation of the issues. Students may have the right to appeal and this is the time when the documentation comes in for scrutiny in relation to all stages being clear and the student having been given appropriate feedback. If the above stages and documentation have been undertaken, then the position is clear, but if for any reason there is doubt about the student having been given appropriate feedback, the panel may well grant the student another attempt.

It is recognized by educational institutions that the role of a mentor is stressful and that advice and support of colleagues in education is necessary in undertaking this role. This takes a variety of forms across the country, but in an attempt to try to strengthen this link the UKCC in the *Fitness for Practice* recommendations has identified the importance of service providers and higher education institutions working together in partnership for all aspects of programmes (UKCC, 1999). In most places this already happens, but there is always room to review this partnership and strengthen aspects of it. There is also a need to review current practices for assessment of learning in practice and identify where the system could be improved. Some suggestions for this are discussed in the conclusion of this chapter.

Future assessment of learning in practice

This chapter has reviewed briefly the many facets of assessing learning in practice, and has provided some practical guidance for those involved in these assessments. Balla and Boyle (1994) discussed the validity of an assessment as being the extent to which the results are meaningful for the assessment purpose they are collected. As practice changes, so do the skills, attitudes and knowledge required by the practitioner. It is for this reason that assessment of learning in practice will continue to be an area of debate and further research.

In a research report about practice and assessment published in 2000, the authors stressed the importance of the assessment criteria being explicit in terms of knowledge, skill, understanding, theory, professional judgement, problem-mapping, and ability to provide rationale for actions (Phillips *et al.*, 2000). Assessment should also be flexible enough to take into account close observation of experience within practice contexts where things do not always remain stable (Fox-Young, 1995, Phillips *et al.*, 2000). Students should continue to have a named mentor but there should be a team-based approach to assessment so that it does not become *ad hoc* in nature and occurs as part of everyday work (Phillips *et al.*, 2000).

All involved in developing these assessments should take this into account and seek new approaches to this essential component of any programme that prepares practitioners for their role in practice. Rowntree (1987) suggested that educators should be more adventurous in the choice of methods used for assessment, and this is perhaps the approach that should taken with assessing learning in practice, where so many variables cannot be taken into account at the time of planning the assessment tool.

References

Andrusyszyn, M A (1989) Clinical evaluation of the effective domain, *Nurse Education Today* **9**, 75–81.

Atkins, M J, Beattie, J and Dockrell, W B (1993) *Assessment Issues in Higher Education*. London: Employment Department Group.

Balla, J and Boyle, P (1994) Assessment of student performance: a framework for improving practice, *Assessment & Evaluation in Higher Education*, **19**(1), 17–28.

Bedford, H, Phillips, T, Robinson, J and Schostak, J (1993) *Assessing Competencies in Nursing and Midwifery Education and Training (Ace Report)*. London: English National Board for Nursing, Midwifery and Health Visiting.

Benner, P (1984) *From Novice to Expert*. Menlo Park, CA: Addison Wesley.

Bondy, K N (1983) Criterion referenced definitions for rating scales in clinical education, *Journal of Nursing Education* **22**(9), 376–81.

Boud, D (1990) Assessment and the promotion of academic values, *Studies in Higher Education*, **15**(1), 101–11.

Bradshaw, A (1997) Defining 'competency' in Nursing (Part 1): a policy review, *Journal of Clinical Nursing*, **6**, 347–54.

Chambers, M A (1998) Some issues in the assessment of clinical practice: a review of the literature, *Journal of Clinical Nursing*, **7**, 201–8.

Coates, V E and Chamber, M (1992) Evaluation of tools to assess clinical competence, *Nurse Education Today*, **12**, 122–9.

Department of Health/English National Board (2001) *Preparation of Mentors and Teachers. A new framework of guidance.* London:DOH/ENB.

English, I (1993) Intuition as a function of the expert nurse: a critique of Benner's novice to expert model, *Journal of Advanced Nursing*, **18**, 387–93.

English National Board for Nursing, Midwifery and Health Visiting (1990) *A New Structure for professional development.* London: ENB.

Fox-Young, S K (1995) Issues in the assessment of expert nurses: purposes, standards and methods, Nurse Education Today, **15**, 96–100.

Gerrish, K (1993) An evaluation of a portfolio as an effective tool for teaching practice placements, *Nurse Education Today*, **13**(3), 172–9.

Girot, E A (2000) Assessment of graduates and diplomats in practice in the UK – are we measuring the same level of competence? *Journal of Clinical Nursing*, **9**, 330–37.

Glen, S and Hight, N F (1992) Portfolios: an effective assessment strategy?, *Nurse Education Today*, **12**(6), 416–23.

Jasper, M A (1995) The potential of a professional portfolio for nursing, *Journal of Clinical Nursing*, **4**, 249–55.

Messick, S (1984) The psychology of educational measurement, *Journal of Educational Measurement*, **21**, 215–38.

Neary, M (1999) Preparing assessors for continuous assessment, *Nursing Standard*, **13**(18), 41–7.

Neary, M (2001) Responsive assessment: assessing student nurses' clinical experience, *Nurse Education Today*, **21**, 3–17.

Newble, D I (1992) Assessing clinical competence at undergraduate level, *Medical Education*, **26**, 504–11.

Nicol, M and Freeth, D (1998) *Assessment of clinical skills: a new approach to an old problem, Nurse Education Today*, **18**, 601–9.

Nicklin, P J and Kenworthy N (2000) Teaching and Assessing in Nursing Practice: an experimental approach, 3rd Edn. London: Bailliere Tindall/Royal College of Nursing.

Nursing & Midwifery Council (2002) Code of Professional Conduct. London: Nursing & Midwifery Council.

Phillips, T, Schostak, J and Tyler, J (2000) *Practice and Assessment in Nursing and Midwifery: doing it for real. Research report series number 16* London: English National Board for Nursing, Midwifery and Health Visiting.

Priest, H and Roberts, P (1998) Assessing student's clinical performance, *Nursing Standard*, **12**(48), 37–41.

Quality Assurance Agency for Higher Education (QAA) (2001) *The framework for higher education qualifications in England, Wales and Northern Ireland.* Gloucester: QAA.

Quinn, F M (2000) *Principles and Practice of Nurse Education*, 4th Edn. Cheltenham: Stanley Thornes.

Rowntree, D (1987) *Assessing students: how shall we know them?* London: Kogan Page.

Toohey, S, Ryan, G and Hughes, C (1996) Assessing the Practicum, *Assessment and Evaluation in Higher Education,* **21**(3), 215–27.

UKCC (1999) *Fitness for Practice,* The UKCC Commission for Nursing and Midwifery Education, chaired by Sir Leonard Peach. London: UKCC.

While, A E (1994) Competence versus performance: which is more important?, *Journal of Advanced Nursing,* **20**, 525–31.

Wood, V (1982) Evaluation of student nurse clinical performance – a continuing performance, *International Nursing Review,* **29**(1), 11–18.

7

Interprofessional Learning in Practice

Scott Reeves and Pam Parker

Introduction

In Chapters 1 and 2 there was reference to the need for students to gain insight into the interprofessional team and all participants' roles. This can be achieved through a variety of strategies, one of which is to develop opportunities for interprofessional practice-based learning. This chapter aims to offer an insight into a range of approaches that can be used by individuals involved in practice-based interprofessional education.[1] It focuses on four factors that help shape this activity: planning processes; learning methods; assessment strategies; and facilitator preparation. To help illuminate the significance of these factors, the chapter discusses both the literature in this area and our experience of developing and evaluating practice-based interprofessional education. Based on this discussion, the chapter goes on to offer a number of 'strategies for success' for individuals involved in this type of education.

Context

There has now been an international enthusiasm for interprofessional education from health policy makers for over two decades (e.g. World Health Organization, 1976; Department of Health and Social Security, 1970; Department of Health, 1989). This enthusiasm has been shared by a number of professional regulatory bodies, including nursing (UKCC, 1999, DOH/ENB, 2001), medicine (GMC, 1993) and social work (CCETSW, 1995). Recently, policy makers in this country re-emphasized their commitment to interprofessional education in their white paper, *A Health Service Of All The Talents*, which outlined the future of education for the health and social care professions (Department of Health, 2000).

At the centre of this policy literature is a belief that this form of learning has the potential to encourage better collaboration between the professions. As a result, interprofessional education has become regarded as an effective approach to improving poor collaboration between health and social care professions, making better use of limited resources and ultimately meeting the complex demands from patients. Barr (2000) offers a detailed understanding of the range of assumptions underpinning this activity (see Figure 7.1).

There has also been a steady growth in reported interprofessional education initiatives over these years. Within the associated literature one can find a variety of different initiatives, from clinical placements for pre-registration students (e.g. Virgin and Goodrow, 1997; Sternas *et al.*,

Interprofessional education facilitates positive interaction
which
engenders mutual understanding and support
which
encourages mutual understanding
which
encourages collaboration between professions
which
spreads the load
which
limits the demands made on any one profession
which
reduces stress
which
enhances job satisfaction
which
improves staff recruitment and retention
which
benefits the professions themselves
which
improves patient care.

Figure 7.1 Underlying assumptions of interprofessional education
[*Source*: Barr (2000)]

1999) to post-registration team-building workshops (e.g. Long, 1996, Latimer *et al.*, 1998).

However, introducing interprofessional education for pre-registration programmes is fraught with difficulties which make this a complex process. Most pre-registration programmes for nursing and medicine have intakes of between 100 and 200 students. In contrast, occupational therapy and physiotherapy programmes have intakes of only between 20 and 60 students. This immediately creates logistical difficulties in finding a suitable location of this type of education. In addition, different intake dates for these student cohorts can create further problems with finding a suitable starting-point for the interprofessional initiative. Obtaining approval from each of the participating professions' regulatory bodies often adds complications, as does agreeing issues of accountability and the financial arrangements that underpin any interprofessional initiative. Given these complexities, it is therefore unsurprising to discover that findings from an ongoing review of interprofessional education have revealed that around two-thirds of reported initiatives occurred after registration (Koppel *et al.*, 2001). In contrast, establishing an interprofessional initiative in this setting is far less problematic. Often, post-registration interprofessional education is an informal activity that occurs during regular team meetings (e.g. Freeth *et al.*, 1999).

Evaluations of interprofessional education indicate that this type of activity can produce a number of positive effects. For example, interprofessional education has been found to address negative attitudes (e.g. Parsell *et al.*, 1998), to develop a better understanding of the other professionals' roles (e.g. Richardson and Edwards, 1997) and to prepare students for interprofessional teamwork (e.g. Virgin *et al.*, 1996). Indeed, findings from recent reviews of interprofessional education have reported that this type of activity can enhance both interprofessional collaboration and make a positive impact on patient care (Koppel *et al.*, 2001; Reeves forthcoming). However, this form of education can also encounter a number of problems. For example, it has been found that staff and students can feel threatened by this type of activity and can resist attempts to introduce it (Freeth *et al.*, 1999); there can be problems with achieving balanced student numbers (Hughes and Lucas, 1997), and difficulties in overcoming poor communication between educational providers (Reeves and Pryce, 1998).

Additionally, there is some debate on identifying the most 'effective' time to introduce interprofessional education to learners. Some authors argue that pre-registration interprofessional education will be more helpful in limiting the processes of negative professional socialization (Parsell and Bligh 1998). Other authors maintain that post-qualification is better as a participant's professional identity is by then formed and so they can link this type of learning directly to their clinical work (Pirrie *et al.*, 1998).

Guiding principles

Having sketched a number of contextual details relating to interprofessional education, we now explore the guiding principles on which this activity is founded.

Interprofessional education is generally founded upon adult learning principles (Barr and Shaw, 1995). Often, initiatives also draw upon work from the fields of social psychology, group learning and psychodynamic theory (Barr and Shaw, 1995, Barr *et al.*, 2000).

To maximize the potential for interprofessional education, Barr (1996, p. 344) argues that interactive learning processes need to be employed to encourage learners so that 'each becomes a resource for the others'. Barr goes on to provide a typology of interactive learning methods that can be used to foster collaboration (see Figure 7.2).

As a consequence of the demand for interactive learning approaches, Barr (1996) points out that staff–student ratios for interprofessional education need to be generous. In the short term, therefore, the cost of this form of education is high. However, over the longer term, it is argued that interprofessional education should pay off in terms of producing more effective collaborative practice which impacts positively on patient care (Barr *et al.*, 1999).

- Exchange-based learning (e.g. debates, role plays)
- Observation-based learning (e.g. work shadowing, joint home visits)
- Action-based learning (e.g. collaborative enquiry, joint research)
- Simulation-based learning (e.g. experiential group work)
- Practice-based learning (e.g. work-related placements)

Figure 7.2   Typology of interprofessional education
[*Source*: Barr (1996)]

Supporting interprofessional education in practice

This section focuses on four key factors that help define interprofessional education in practice: planning processes; learning methods; assessment strategies; and facilitator preparation. We draw on the literature and on our experience in developing and evaluating practice-based interprofessional education.

Planning processes

Before attempting to deliver any form of practice-based interprofessional education, attention should be paid to the planning process. As any interprofessional initiative involves merging different professional groups, with different educational and practical needs and demands effective planning is required.

Planning issues

For Casto (1994) one of the most crucial parts of the planning process is to ensure that senior management commitment is obtained from all participating organizations. Without this type of commitment, access to resources (e.g. teaching equipment) needed for an interprofessional initiative cannot usually be secured.

In addition, finance needs careful consideration during the planning of any interprofessional initiative. As the cost of this form of education tends to 'span many professional budgets' (Goble 1994, p. 177), agreement over financial arrangements can often be a main hurdle for interprofessional education. For LaSala *et al.* (1997) this issue was resolved when they secured external funding to cover the costs of their interprofessional course for pre-registration nursing, social work and health administrator students. However, it is rare to secure funding to plan and implement interprofessional education.

Another factor to consider is the membership of the planning group. As developing this type of education can take considerable time and energy, Lary *et al.* (1997) argue that group members need to have a high level of dedication. This was certainly the case in our work of planning and evaluating an interprofessional clinical placement for nursing, medical, occupational therapy and physiotherapy students. We found that it was only through the sustained enthusiasm of steering group members, who overcame various practical issues such as adjustments to programmes and time, that a pilot placement was established. Without this type of group effort, interprofessional education cannot be developed and implemented; further information on this initiative can be found in Freeth and Reeves (1999), Freeth *et al.* (2001), Reeves *et al.* (forthcoming). Our experience of developing and evaluating practice-based interprofessional initiatives over a number of years has also been helpful in developing a series of suggestions for groups beginning the process of planning for a practice-based interprofessional initiative. First, there should be equal representation of the different groups involved in the initiative. This helps to ensure that no one group can dominate the planning process and skew the initiative in any one direction. Second, group members need to share their aims and assumptions about the initiative to ensure that all members are working towards a common goal. Where differences are identified, these need to be discussed and resolved. Third, regular planning meetings should be held to allow group members to update one another and jointly solve any difficulties they encounter in the planning process. Finally, the selection of a project leader may be helpful in coordinating the activities of the group and encouraging progress to ensure that planning processes are effective.

Learning methods

As noted above, a range of possible interactive learning methods is available. In considering this issue in further depth we examine the use of different learning methods within practice-based interprofessional education.

Target the learning

When selecting learning methods care is required to ensure that they are suitable for the potential learning needs of group. For example, Miller *et al.* (1999) argue that inexperienced pre-registration learners should be offered activities focused on developing communication skills and understanding one another's professional roles to allow them to develop initial insights into the concepts that underpin collaboration. However, qualified practitioners should be offered more experiential learning focused around developing strategies for teamwork that they can actually apply to their practice. Hilton *et al.* (1995) offer a similar approach to targeting interprofessional education (see Table 7.1). Using this approach, level 1 could be helpfully employed for pre-registration learners and level 2 for qualified practitioners.

Table 7.1   Team development

Knowledge	Skills	Attitudes
Level 1 Develop inter- disciplinary awareness	Communicate with other healthcare professionals	Appreciate inter- disciplinary team care
Understand roles of other professions		Accept that opinions of colleagues are as vital as their own
Level 2 Identify areas of unique responsibility for each member of the team and areas of overlap	Participate actively in cooperative goal structuring in relation to patient care	Value the opinions of colleagues Be willing to give, receive and share information
	Collaborate and negotiate with colleagues	Appreciate that complex client problems demand an interdisciplinary approach
	Work collaboratively within a multi- disciplinary health care team	

Source: Adapted from Hilton *et al.* (1995)

'*Breaking the ice*'

When a group comes together to undertake interprofessional learning for the first time, attention should be paid to the initial process of group formation. The use of an 'ice-breaking' session is considered helpful in facilitating group cohesion (e.g. Sternas *et al.*, 1999). Ice-breaking sessions allow learners to focus interactively on professional stereotyping or professional assumptions they bring to an interprofessional initiative. This type of learning activity is particularly advantageous in unpacking and exploring issues of professionalism (e.g. boundary protectionism) that are central to any collaborative venture. They are also helpful in team-building, especially when a group of learners have not previously worked together. For established interprofessional teams these sessions can also be useful in allowing these teams to unpack issues linked to hierarchy and power differentials that surround their daily practice (Hugman, 1991).

Combining learning methods

In order to provide interprofessional education that is both stimulating and interesting, a variety of different interactive learning methods should be employed. For example, Virgin and Goodrow (1997) incorporated interprofessional discussions for nursing, medical and social work students and also a team-based problem-solving activity called the 'community crossword', where students collected information from patients and community-based services. Similarly, in an evaluation undertaken by one of us (Reeves *et al.*, 2000) of an interprofessional initiative designed to enhance collaboration between newly qualified nurses and doctors, the use of joint discussion, scenario-based problem-solving and shared hands-on clinical activities were considered helpful in fostering the skills and knowledge that underpin collaboration. Combining learning activities during an interprofessional initiative may also achieve a more profound level of learning. For example, the use of seminar-based discussions with practice-based learning can help underpin experiential practice-based learning with more conceptual input gained from classroom sessions. In our work in developing and evaluating an interprofessional clinical placement for teams of nursing, medical, occupational therapy and physiotherapy students (e.g. Freeth and Reeves, 1999; Reeves *et al.*, 2001), it was found that the use of interactive classroom activities such as group reflection sessions aided the students' interprofessional teamwork skills. In particular, students reported that leaving the clinical learning environment to spend time reflecting upon their experiences deepened their understanding of the issues and process of interprofessional team work.

Informal learning

Opportunities for informal learning (e.g. when learners meet socially to discuss aspects of their formal education) are a useful approach for practice-based interprofessional education. For Bond (1997) informal learning is helpful in allowing individuals to exchange ideas and obtain guidance from their peers, work colleagues or managers.

Informal learning activities can be explicitly built into an interprofessional programme. O'Boyle *et al.* (1995), for example, describe how course organizers ensured that all the learners in an interprofessional initiative had the opportunity to share time when eating their lunch which encouraged them to discuss their education informally. Informal learning can also occur as an 'unplanned' outcome of an interprofessional initiative. In an evaluation one of us undertook (Reeves, 2000) it was found that nursing, medical and dental students on a community-based module used pubs and cafés after their formal learning sessions to discuss and reflect upon their interprofessional learning informally. For these students, this type of learning was felt to be a valuable part of their shared experiences on this module. In particular, these informal learning opportunities allowed the students to consolidate and enrich the experiences gained from the formal learning on the module.

Possible problems

It should be recognized that a number of potential problems can arise with the use of interactive learning methods in interprofessional education. For example, Itano *et al.* (1991) found that allowing learners 'space' for interaction, especially when problem solving, can mean that groups experience friction linked to defending their different professional approaches. (Where friction does arise within teams, it should be used creatively by facilitators to explore the various professional issues that underpin collaboration. Facilitation of interprofessional groups is considered later in the chapter.)

Combining learning activities designed to promote *collaborative* outcomes with those designed to promote more *profession-specific* outcomes can be problematic. As Fallsberg and Wijma (1999) found, learners experience uncertainty about the overall aim of the interprofessional education. This issue emerged during our work on the interprofessional placement for nursing, medical, occupational therapy and physiotherapy students (Freeth and Reeves, 1999; Freeth *et al.*, 2001). In order to give students a holistic insight into a clinical environment, they were offered both collaborative interactive learning activities such as team problem solving and profession-specific activities such as drug administration (a task that the nursing students exclusively undertook). For the students on this placement, the inclusion of both collaborative and profession-specific learning activities produced tension, as it was found difficult to participate actively in both. After feeding this finding back to the group responsible for developing the placement, it has been agreed to review this part of the placement in an attempt to reduce this tension.

In post-registration initiatives, one has to be aware that learning activities can be affected by the demands of clinical work, especially if sessions are held near the learners' clinical area. This difficulty was experienced when running interprofessional education sessions for newly qualified nurses and doctors. In particular, it was found that doctors were frequently being bleeped (usually on non-urgent business). This interrupted the processes of group learning. In an attempt to overcome this problem in future, it has been decided to ensure that the doctors leave their bleep with a person who can screen calls. One way of overcoming this difficulty is to offer clinical teams residential interprofessional education. This type of course can be rewarding in terms of providing a far more conducive learning environment for interprofessional learning (Long, 1996). It can also provide ample opportunity for important processes of informal learning (Latimer *et al.*, 1998). However, it is an expensive option, especially as one needs to secure clinical cover for the team.

Assessment

Careful consideration needs to be given to the type of learning assessment employed for practice-based interprofessional education. As with any educational activity, the choice of assessment of learning can significantly affect both the learning processes and outcomes.

Formative assessment

Typically, assessment of learning on practice-based interprofessional education is formative. There are a number of reasons why this is the case. As previously noted, in pre-registration initiatives, problems can often be encountered in aligning different requirements of professional validation bodies for the different groups of students. For example, in our work on an interprofessional clinical placement for nursing, medical, occupational therapy and physiotherapy students, the differing requirements of professional registration from the four regulatory bodies meant that this placement could not offer a summative assessment for the participating students, as it was a pilot study. Clearly, this lack of 'formal' assessment may diminish learner motivation for interprofessional education. However, the evaluation of this initiative revealed that this issue did not have a significant effect on the students' overall enjoyment of their practice-based interprofessional learning (Freeth and Reeves, 1999). Similarly, in other work one of us has undertaken (Reeves, 2000) the process of learning together with colleagues from other professional groups appears to outweigh potential problems with student motivation.

Assessment is often further complicated because meeting the different requirements of the professional validation bodies can result in pre-registration initiatives using different types of learning assessment between student groups. However, as Sternas *et al.* (1999) found, where they assessed students differently (nursing students needed to complete an essay, medical students had no such assessment), differing levels of student enthusiasm were encountered. As post-registration practice-based interprofessional education tends to emerge in response to overcoming a problem with service delivery (e.g. Horak *et al.*, 1991; Heil *et al.*, 1997; Young *et al.*, 1998), there is usually no rationale for undertaking a summative assessment. Any assessment of interprofessional learning in these areas is normally linked to reported improvements in working practices and delivery of care to patients. However, there are a handful of formal post-registration courses where summative assessment of interprofessional education is offered to learners (e.g. Stubblefield *et al.*, 1994; Reader *et al.*, 1999).

Possible approaches

The literature offers a range of approaches to assessing practice-based interprofessional education. These include: development of multidisciplinary care plans (Brown and Adkins, 1989); team presentations of approaches to care (Itano *et al.*, 1991); end-of-session feedback (Swanson *et al.*, 1998); and written assignment relating to process of delivering interprofessional care (Bezzina *et al.*, 1998).

It is often advantageous to combine a team presentation with an individual written assignment to assess both learners' teamwork skills and individual knowledge of collaboration. This was the approach taken in the community module for nursing, medical and dental students that one of us evaluated (Reeves and Pryce, 1998). In this module, poster presentations were used to assess the student teams' knowledge of community care and individual diaries were used to assess the students' insight into the processes of teamwork.

In post-registration education, where time can be more limited, assessments of learning need to be adapted to reflect these restrictions. For example, in the interprofessional sessions for newly qualified nurses and doctors that one of us evaluated (Reeves *et al.*, 2000), learning was assessed by use of verbal feedback from interprofessional group discussions of clinical scenarios. In this initiative, given time was short (the sessions had a two-hour duration), this type of learning assessment was considered the most realistic.

Facilitator preparation

Lecturers need to be well prepared to meet the demands of facilitating interprofessional groups as this type of facilitation is more often demanding than their traditional work with a group made up only of nursing learners. Interprofessional facilitators need to pay attention to group dynamics (e.g. handling issues related to professional socialization and boundary protectionism) while ensuring that opportunities for practice-based learning within the group are maximized. In addition, facilitators need to ensure that all learners have an equal input into the interprofessional group-work while guarding against adversely affecting the group learning processes they are facilitating.

Where no preparation is offered, it is found that staff encounter problems with the rigours of facilitating interprofessional groups. For example, in an evaluation that one of us undertook (Reeves *et al.*, 2000), it was found that one facilitator tended to dominate one group. This inhibited discussion and interprofessional problem solving. As a result of this finding, it has been agreed by the course organizers to offer facilitators some initial input into their work with these interprofessional groups of staff nurses and junior doctors.

Facilitator expertise

In order to manage the demands that interprofessional education makes of a facilitator, the literature (e.g. Funnell, 1995;, Hammick, 1998) suggests a range of attributes that are required for this type of work. These include:

- experience of interprofessional work (to draw upon when facilitating);
- in-depth understanding of interactive learning methods;
- knowledge of group dynamics;
- confidence in working with interprofessional groups; and
- flexibility (to creatively use professional differences within groups).

Barr (1996, p. 244) draws together these varying attributes when he states that the interprofessional facilitator needs 'to be attuned to the dynamics of interprofessional learning, skilled in optimising learning opportunities, valuing the distinctive experience and expertise which each of the participating professions brings'.

Training

Clearly, the above attributes are not easy to acquire. Therefore formal preparation may need to be considered. However, there appears to be only a limited number of courses for facilitators. From a search of the literature only three courses could be located: two in the UK (Moseley, 1997, Mhaolrúnaigh and Clifford, 1998) and one in the US (Clay *et al.*, 1999). Encouragingly, all appear to offer a similar type of input, focusing on understanding the different professions' roles and responsibilities, exploring issues of professionalism and planning learning strategies for interprofessional groups.[2]

Where formal training cannot be obtained, it is advisable to seek informal input from a colleague more experienced in this type of work. Often, it is useful to consider team teaching with more experienced colleagues to help develop the range of necessary skills, knowledge and confidence that are vital for interprofessional facilitation.

Strategies for success

The chapter concludes by drawing together the discussion and offering a number of strategies for success in the three areas considered.

Planning processes

To ensure that practice-based interprofessional education is well planned, care should be paid to the following:

- Senior management support for the initiative needs to be obtained before any initiative can be developed.
- Agreeing shared financing of interprofessional initiatives can be difficult. Therefore careful negotiation is needed.
- As considerable time and energy are spent planning an interprofessional initiative, group members need to have a high level of dedication.
- To achieve smooth teamwork within the planning group, team processes need to be considered.

Learning methods

To ensure appropriate learning methods are employed within practice-based interprofessional education, attention needs to be paid to the following:

- To make learning relevant, target the different learning methods for the stage in the development of the interprofessional group.

- Employ a range of interactive learning activities to keep interprofessional education lively and stimulating.
- Underpin experiential learning with conceptual learning to offer a more profound understanding of the practices and theories of interprofessional collaboration.
- Use ice-breaking activities to help unpack issues around their professional socialization and possible boundary protectionism.
- Be aware of the problems that can arise with practice-based interprofessional education. Be creative in overcoming these problems.

Assessment

To encourage effective assessment of learning within practice-based interprofessional education care should be paid to the following:

- Summative assessment of learning can be problematic for pre-registration education, or unnecessary for post-registration education. Formative assessment may be more a useful approach for interprofessional education.
- Be consistent when assessing student learning as uneven assessment can affect motivation.
- Carefully consider the range of learning assessments that can be used in interprofessional education.
- Combine different learning assessments to understand the impact of interprofessional education on team and individual learning.
- Be realistic with assessment strategies, especially in post-registration education where time for learning is usually more restricted.

Facilitator preparation

In providing adequate preparation of facilitators for practice-based interprofessional education attention needs to be paid to the following:

- Interprofessional facilitation is a difficult task. Poor facilitation can adversely affect student learning. Therefore facilitators require a high level of preparation in group dynamics and group learning processes.
- Where formal preparation for interprofessional facilitation cannot be obtained, informal input from more experienced colleagues could be used.

Notes

1   There continues to be uncertainty about the definition of 'interprofessional education'. In this chapter, we employ the term 'interprofessional education' based upon the following definition: occasions when two or more professions learn together with the object of cultivating collaborative practice (Barr, 1996 p. 347).

2   Information on current UK-based facilitator training can be obtained by contacting The Centre For the Advancement of Interprofessional Education (www.caipe.org.uk).

References

Barr, H (1996) Ends to means in interprofessional education: towards a typology, *Education for Health*, **9**, 341–52.

Barr, H (2000) *Interprofessional Education 1997–2000: A Review*. London: CAIPE.

Barr, H & Shaw, I (1995) *Shared Learning: Selected Examples from the Literature*. London: CAIPE.

Barr, H, Freeth, D, Hammick, M, Koppel, I and Reeves, S (2000) *Evaluations of Interprofessional Education: A United Kingdom Review for Health and Social Care*. London: CAIPE.

Barr, H, Hammick, M, Koppel, I an& Reeves, S (1999) Evaluating interprofessional education: two reviews for health and social care, *British Educational Research Journal*, **25**, 533–44.

Bezzina, P, Keogh, J and Keogh, M (1998) Teaching primary health care: an interdisciplinary approach, *Nurse Education Today*, **18**, 36–45.

Bond, M (1997) A learning team in the making, *Journal of Interprofessional Care*, **11**, 89–98.

Brown, V and Adkins, B (1989) A comprehensive training program for multi-disciplinary treatment plans, *Journal of Nursing Staff Development*, **5**, 25–9.

Casto, M (1994) Education for interprofessional practice. In Casto, M and Julia, M (eds), *Interprofessional Care and Collaborative Practice*. Belmont: Brooks/Cole.

CCETSW (1995) *Assuring Quality in the Diploma in Social Work. Rules and requirements for the DipSW*. London: Central Council for Education and Training in Social Work.

Clay, M, Lilley, S, Borre, K and Harris, J (1999) Applying adult education principles to the design of a preceptor development program, *Journal of Interprofessional Care*, **13**, 405–15.

Department of Health (1989) *Caring for People. Community Care in the Next Decade*. London: HMSO.

Department of Health (2000) *Consultative Document: A Health Service Of All The Talents: Developing the NHS Workforce*. London: DOH.

Department of Health/English National Board (2001) *Placements in Focus: Guidance for Education in Practice for Health Care Professions.* London: DOH/ENB.

Department of Health and Social Security (1970) *Report of the Committee on Local Authority and Allied Personal Social Services.* London: HMSO.

Fallsberg, M and Wijma K (1999*)* Student attitudes towards the goals of an interprofessional training ward,. *Medical Teacher*, **6**, 576–81.

Freeth, D, Meyer, J, Reeves, S and Spilsbury, K (1999*)* Linking interprofessional education to user benefit: of drops in the ocean and stalactites, *Advancing Clinical Nursing*, **3**, 127–35.

Freeth, D and Reeves, S (1999) *Interprofessional Training Ward Pilot Phase: Evaluation Project Report.* London: City University Internal Research Report.

Freeth, D, Reeves, S, Goreham, C, Parker, P, Haynes S and Pearson, S (2001) 'Real life' clinical learning on an interprofessional training ward, *Nurse Education Today*, **21**, 366–72.

Funnell, P (1995) Exploring the value of interprofessional shared learning. In Soothill, K, Mackay, L and Webb, C (eds), *Interprofessional Relations in Health Care.* London: Edward Arnold.

GMC (1993) *Tomorrow's Doctors.* London: General Medical Council.

Goble, R (1994) Multiprofessional education in Europe: an overview. In Leathard, A (ed.), *Going Interprofessional: Working Together for Health and Welfare.* London: Routledge.

Hammick, M (1998) Interprofessional education: concept, theory and application, *Journal of Interprofessional Care*, **12**, 323–32.

Heil, R, Lane, S, Maahs, D, Miner, J, Myers, C and Roth, J (1997) Using a performance improvement team to reinvent a mandatory education program, *Joint Commission Journal on Quality Improvement*, **23**, 103–16.

Hilton, R, Morris, D and Wright, A (1995) Learning to work in the heath care team, *Journal of Interprofessional Care*, **9**, 167–74.

Horak, B, Guarino, J, Knight, C and Kweder, S (1991) Building a team on a medical floor, *Health Care Management Review*, **16**, 65–71.

Hughes, L and Lucas, J (1997) An evaluation of problem based learning in the multiprofessional education curriculum for the health professions, *Journal of Interprofessional Care*, **11**, 77–88.

Hugman, R (1991) *Power in the Caring Professions.* London: Macmillan.

Itano, J, Williams, J, Deaton, M and Oishi N (1991) Impact of a student interdisciplinary oncology team project, *Journal of Cancer Education*, **6**, 219–26.

Koppel, I, Barr, H, Reeves, S, Freeth, D and Hammick, M (2001) Establishing a systematic approach to evaluating the effectiveness of interprofessional education. *Issues in Interdisciplinary Care*, **3**, 41–9.

Lary, M, Lavigne, S, Muma, S, Jones, S and Hoeft, H (1997) Breaking down barriers: multidisciplinary education model', *Journal of Allied Health*, Spring, 63–9.

LaSala, K, Hopper, S, Rissmeyer, D and Shipe, D (1997) Rural health care & interdisciplinary education, *Nursing and Health Care Perspectives*, **18**, 292–8.

Latimer, E, Kiehl, K, Lennox, S and Studd, S (1998) An interdisciplinary palliative care course for practising health professionals: ten years' experience,
Journal of Palliative Care, **14**, 27–33.

Long, S (1996) Primary health care team workshop: team members' perspectives, *Journal of Advanced Nursing*, **23**, 935–41.

Mhaolrúnaigh, S and Clifford, C (1998) The preparation of teachers for shared
learning environments, *Nurse Education Today*, **18**, 178–82.

Miller, C, Ross, N and Freeman, M (1999) *Shared Learning and Clinical Teamwork:
New Directions in Education for Multiprofessional Teams*. London: ENB.

Moseley, M (1997) Teaching the teachers: the East Anglian interprofessional
practice teaching programmes at the University of East Anglia, *CAIPE
Bulletin*, **13**, 23–4.

O'Boyle, M, Paniagua, F, Wassef, A and Holzer, C (1995) Training health
professionals in the recognition and treatment of depression, *Psychiatric
Services*, **46**, 616–18.

Parsel,l G and Bligh J (1998) Educational principles underpinning successful
shared learning, *Medical Teacher*, **20**, 522–9.

Parsel,l G, Spalding, R and Bligh, J (1998) Shared goals, shared learning: evaluation of a multiprofessional course for undergraduate students, *Medical
Education*, **32**, 304–11.

Pirrie, A, Wilson, V, Harden, R and Elsegood, J (1998) AMEE Guide No. 12:
Multiprofessional education part 2 – promoting cohesive practice in health
care, *Medical Teacher*, **20**, 409–16.

Reader, F, Hunt, K, Passmore, H, Royce,S and Adapa, U (1999) Professional
development in reproductive and sexual health—a pilot study from Suffolk,
UK *British Journal of Family Planning*, **24**, 135–40.

Reeves, S (forthcoming) A review of the effects of Interprofessional education on
staff involved in the care of adults with mental health problems, *Journal of
Psychiatric and Mental Health Nursing*.

Reeves, S (2000) Community-based interprofessional education for medical,
nursing and dental students, *Health and Social Care in the Community*, **8**, 269–76.

Reeves, S, Freeth, D, McCrorie, P and Perry D (forthcoming) 'It teaches you
what to expect in real life' interprofessional education on a training ward for
medical, nursing, occupational therapy and physiotherapy students, *Medical
Education*.

Reeves, S, Freeth, D, Nicol, M and Wood, D (2000) A joint learning venture
between new nurses and junior doctors, Nursing Times, **96**(38), 39–40.

Reeves, S and Pryce, A. (1998) Emerging Themes: an exploratory research
project of a multidisciplinary education module for medical, dental and nursing students, *Nurse Education Today*, **18**, 534–41.

Richardson, J and Edwards, M (1997) An undergraduate clinical skills laboratory developing interprofessional skills in physical and occupational therapy,
Gerontology and Geriatrics Education, **17**, 33–43.

Sternas, K, O'Hare, P, Lehman, K and Milligan, R (1999) Nursing and medical student teaming for service learning in partnership with the community: an emerging holistic model for interdisciplinary education and practice, *Holistic Nursing Practice*, **12**, 66–77.

Stubblefield, C, Houston, C and Haire, J (1994) Interactive use of models of health-related behavior to promote interdisciplinary collaboration, *Journal of Allied Health*, **23**, 237–43.

Swanson, E, Taylor, C, Valentine, A, and McCarthy, A (1998) The integrated health professions education program seminar, *Nurse Educator*, **23**, 18–21.

UKCC (1999) *Fitness for Practice*, The UKCC Commission for Nursing and Midwifery Education chaired by Sir Leonard Peach. London: UKCC.

Virgin, S and Goodrow, B (1997) A community crossword puzzle. An interdisciplinary approach to community-based learning, *Nursing and Health Care Perspectives*, **18**, 302–7.

Virgin, S, Goodrow, B and Duggins, B (1996) Scavenger hunt: a community-based learning experience, *Nurse Educator*, **21**, 32–4.

Young, M, Gooder, V, Oltermann, M, Bohman, C, French, T and James, B (1998) The impact of a multidisciplinary approach on caring for ventilator-dependent patients, *International Journal for Quality in Health Care*, **10**, 15–26.

World Health Organisation (1976) *Continuing Education of Health Personnel*. Copenhagen: WHO Regional Office for Europe.

8

Providing Educator Support for Practice Learning

Maggie Mallik and Liz Aston

Introduction

In Chapters 1, 2 and 3 the link lecturer's role and the need for support have been outlined. The key to successful practice-based learning is to ensure that students in the healthcare professions are provided with a 'scaffolding' of structured support (Quality Support Centre, 1995a–e; Quality Assurance Agency, 2001). It is accepted in the UK that the majority of support is currently delivered through practitioner–student partnerships in practice environments that are conducive to learning. Increasingly patients/clients, especially those people who are confident in managing their own healthcare needs, are becoming more actively involved in the learning partnerships.

Although formal responsibility for the quality of an education programme rests with the Higher Education Institute (HEI), courses that concurrently prepare students for a professional qualification with registration need considerable input to learners from qualified practitioners. However, for healthcare practitioners, tensions do exist between the need to provide a quality service to patients/clients and the demands made on them in teaching and assessing an increasing numbers of healthcare learners. It is important therefore to debate how support from an educator, that is, a teacher/lecturer, can influence the effectiveness of practice-based learning.

Recent policy documents (UKCC, 1999; DOH, 1999, 2000) have

highlighted the need for effective partnerships between health service providers and HEIs in facilitating the provision of good-quality structured support for all learners in practice placements. In response to these strategy drivers, new models for practice learning support are being developed in the UK. This chapter aims to review past and current models of formalized teacher/lecturer support for practice learning and explore in more detail two new initiatives in the UK instigated through innovative partnerships between NHS Trusts and HEIs.

Before reviewing past and current models of provision of support for practice learning, it is important to clarify the nature of that learning. In providing teacher support in a practice environment, the student is always viewed as an active participant. The model of 'cognitive apprenticeship' advocated by Taylor and Dean Care (1999) best describes the current role of student nurses in healthcare placements in the UK. Although supernumerary, they are active participants and continue to learn through the apprenticeship mode of observing, being coached by an expert, and practising. They not only gain explicit knowledge and skills in communication, psychomotor and clinical decision making, but also need to develop the processes of integrating the knowledge with the conditions under which that knowledge applies and the culture in which that knowledge is used (Eraut, 1999). Expert practitioners acting as mentors are recognized to have the key role in practice learning.

With a belief in the cognitive apprenticeship model of practice learning, the role of the lecturer/practice educator is not one of primarily providing discrete teaching activity, but the much broader roles of facilitation of learning and of developing the learning environment. In this model, effective teaching methods must have the capacity to externalize the largely internal knowledge and thought processes underpinning clinical practice. Collins *et al.* (1989) include multiple methods for doing this, such as role modelling, coaching, scaffolding, articulating, reflecting and exploration. Along with organizing the appropriate sequencing of learning experiences and exploring the influence of context and culture on practice learning, lecturers/practice educators have a developmental and supportive role in practice learning. Their partnerships with practitioners provide the 'scaffold' needed for quality work-based learning.

Past provision

Historically, training for the nursing profession was completed through the traditional apprenticeship mode. Students learned about nursing by participating in practice over long periods of time. Learning by 'doing' was the dominant model with the practice expert, the ward sister having the strongest influence on student learning (Orton, 1982; Ogier, 1981; Fretwell, 1982). Schools of nursing provided preparation, with detailed attention to learning the practical skills of the professional role in the safe environment of the school practical room. Examinations included both theory and practice elements of the curriculum. Practical demonstrations and oral questioning were the norm, with control centralized through the national syllabus provided by governing bodies such as the General Nursing Council (GNC). The title given to the teacher, that is, 'Sister Tutor', demonstrated the cultural influence of the ward sister in the school setting. Wearing the nurse's uniform in the classroom added to the ambience of the strong practice influence on training methods. The dominant influence of the ward sister role began to wane in the late 1960s as other pressures on their time reduced their educational role.

The clinical teacher

A new role of clinical teacher was introduced through clinical teaching courses provided by the Royal College of Nursing (RCN), beginning in 1958. Formal status and training meant that the unique skills of teaching in a clinical environment were recognized. Qualified practitioners completed a recommended six-month full-time course in order to register as clinical teachers. Numbers appointed and interpretation of the role was variable. Although initially valued, the role was not a complete success and due to numerous problems was eventually phased out in the mid-1980s (ENB, 1985).

The main problems with the clinical teacher role are attributed by research studies and anecdotal evidence to the tensions arising out of the combination of the two roles of 'nurse' and 'teacher' (Kirkwood, 1979; Robertson, 1987; Martin, 1989). There was lack of understanding of the role by both clinical and tutorial staff. Dissatisfaction with the job arose from the relatively low status of the clinical teacher in the school hierarchy and their corresponding lack of authority and power to influence policy decision making in the practice setting. Many clinical teachers moved on to the higher-status job of 'nurse tutor' as soon as possible. *The Salmon Report* (Ministry of Health, 1966) had already acknowledged that these posts were seen as a way into education and were used to test the nurse's aptitude for teaching. However, it is interesting to note that data collected from experienced practitioners at the end of the 1990s (Day *et al.*, 1998) referred to the clinical teacher role as being a positive experience for them as students. These practitioners, given current work pressures, were now requesting that clinical teacher roles needed to be re-created. Overall it should be noted that there was relatively little systematic study completed on the impact or effectiveness of the clinical teacher post apart from the descriptive work completed by Kirkwood (1979), Roberston (1987) and Martin (1989).

The apparent failure of the clinical teaching post to have any impact on the theory–practice gap or to produce stability and job satisfaction for the incumbents led to the phasing out of the six-month courses provided for this post in the mid-1980s. At this time the importance of the practitioner providing clinical teaching was re-emphasized through the establishment of mentorship schemes, the focus on continuous assessment of practice as opposed to 'one-off assessments' and the instigation of teaching and assessing courses such as the English National Board (ENB) course number 998, and The City and Guilds 730/7307. Recommendations that senior nursing posts should require a teaching and assessing qualification became the norm. Although there have been problems with the standard and quality of these preparation programmes (Philips *et al.*, 1994; Neary, 1999), they continued to be a required qualification for practitioners undertaking supervisory roles up to the year 2000. New mentorship preparation programmes, which follow guidelines set by the UK Nursing and Midwifery Council, are now being instigated by the HEIs (DOH/ENB, 2001; UKCC, 2000).

Current models

With the formalized phasing out of the clinical tTeacher role in the mid-1980s, it was re-emphasized in the late 1980s that nurse tutors still had a role to play in practice education and now became responsible for clinical teaching as well as classroom work. Teacher preparation courses approved by the professional boards were to include a component that would prepare teachers for their role in practice, and the recommendation that up to 20 per cent of teaching time should be spent in the practice setting became the expected standard (ENB, 1989, 1995). The assimilation of nurse education into higher education in the mid 1990s-did not change the obligation on teachers/lecturers to provide support for students in the practice setting (ENB, 1997). The most common term used to describe the role is that of 'link lecturer' (Day *et al.*, 1998).

Link lecturer support

Lecturer support within the practice-learning environment has a history of ambiguity in how the role is both interpreted and realized within practice. Varied interpretations lead to considerable difficulty in determining the purpose of the role, with lack of clarity leading to difficulty in developing standards. Criteria for an evaluation of the effectiveness of the role are difficult to achieve (Day *et al.*, 1998; Watson and Harris, 1999). This results in a potentially valuable role not being developed and supported by the HEI. Rationalization of expenditure in university departments and the competitive nature of contracting to provide cost-effective education in nursing and midwifery throughout the 1990s meant that time for practice teaching was viewed as an expensive luxury. Lecturer time spent in supporting practice learning needs evidence of effectiveness in order to justify investing valuable resources.

The expectation that all teachers of nursing should spend a proportion of their time in clinical teaching and/or in a role that would provide support for practice learning has led to considerable variety in the application of this requirement. Numerous studies, completed up to the end of the 1990s, have highlighted problems for teachers/lecturers fulfilling this component of their role (White *et al.*, 1993; Clifford, 1993; Luker *et al.*, 1995; Day *et al.*, 1998). The dominant feature is that university lecturers do not have time to fulfil the role and it is given low priority at an individual and organizational level.

Numerous interpretations of how the role should be fulfilled have added to the confusion. There is a perceived lack of effectiveness, particularly recognized by students and practitioners (Day *et al.*, 1998). A variety of activities are undertaken within the role, with the dominant model being that of linking or liaising with the practice setting. HEIs have a standard that all placements areas should, at the very least, have a named lecturer contact. With the integration of colleges of nursing into HEIs in the mid-1990s, the potential for role tensions to be compounded by the extra demands of academic credibility through research and publication has been verified (Luker *et al.*, 1995; Day *et al.*, 1998).

Lecturers, students and practitioners can see the potential value of lecturers providing support for practice learning. However, rhetoric about the value of the role does not always match the reality (MacNeil, 1997). Lecturers tend to feel guilty about lack of prioritization of time for the role, which may be due to their workload, perceived lack of clinical expertise, confusion about role expectations, numbers of placements they are responsible for and how valued they feel when they visit place-ments. Practitioners reinforce this ambivalence, as they do not always welcome lecturer involvement. It can sometimes appear to be an 'inspec-tor' role, viewed as checking and monitoring the practitioner's perfor-mance rather than helping to facilitate and support the practitioner's role in teaching students.

Students in addition expect support in practice to be given a high priority, but the reality is that experiences of lecturer support are vari-able, with contact usually being on an *ad hoc* basis. They expect regular, pre-planned visits, where their progress can be discussed. Preferably this should include the mentor, with lecturers having some input to the assessment process in order to ensure objectivity within the process (Day *et al.*, 1998). Practitioner views of the lecturer's role reinforce these find-ings, as 'pop in' visits do not allow practitioners the opportunity to focus their thoughts in order to make effective use of their access to the lecturer's time. Developing clear expectations of the role, with systems of support that include regular, structured contact, would enable all parties to use time constructively in terms of developing the learning environ-ment and meeting the needs of students and mentors.

Support requires the visible presence of lecturers within the clinical setting to demonstrate to both students and practitioners that practice truly is valued as part of the educational process and not seen as divorced from the educational experience. The qualities of the lecturer are para-mount here, exceeding in importance qualities such as clinical expertise and competence. The lecturer needs to have both the interpersonal and intrapersonal qualities that facilitate the building of effective relation-ships (Aston *et al.*, 2000). The visibility of lecturers in practice has no value if respect, trust and dialogue are not forthcoming.

Although there are various roles that a lecturer may undertake within practice, such as clinical teacher, practice development, taking a case-load of patients, and research activity, there appears to be a minimum of three main aspects to the role that are necessary for the lecturer to focus upon. These are:

- developing the learning environment;
- supporting the student; and
- supporting the practice mentor.

In developing the learning environment, the lecturer has a pivotal role in assisting the practitioner to review existing learning opportunities and

identify new ones (DOH/ENB, 2001). The lecturer's educational expertise is invaluable in terms of assisting practitioners to structure the
student's learning experience to complement their stage of development,
to support the learning process and to monitor progress. Through academic staff and practitioners working together, both parties can be seen
to be part of a learning organization that can help to minimize the
perception of a theory/practice divide by students.

Placement environments also need to be carefully prepared and
continually developed to ensure the student experiences good-quality
care and treatment of clients, have good role models and see that staff
value learning (DOH/ENB, 2001). Lecturers and practitioners have
joint responsibility for ensuring this occurs in order to encourage the
student to gain the most from their experiences.

For the student, both personal and professional development can be
supported and facilitated through reflection. With regular contact, the
lecturer can help build a climate of trust in which reflection can assist
the student to critique personal and professional assumptions. This can
help the student to 'grow' through questioning the appropriateness of
theoretical principles and their experiences within nursing practice
(Smith, 1998). In addition, reflection can empower the student and helps
to facilitate their development as an independent learner (Hancock,
1999) as, central to 'learning on the job' is the development of an awareness of one's own learning processes.

Becoming a mentor can be one of the greatest challenges a registered
nurse faces (Aston, 2000), and mentors need support from lecturers as
well as peers in order to develop this role effectively. Duffy (2000) states
that mentors require this input from lecturers at placement level.
However, currently there does appear to be a distinct lack of support for
the mentors of students (Aston, 2000). Lecturer support can assist the
mentor in knowing the level at which the student should be and in assisting mentors in their understanding of what is meant by diploma and
degree levels of practice (Luker *et al.*, 1995, White *et al.*, 1993).

The mentor's assessmentr role also creates concern and anxiety,
particularly if there is little feedback to the assessor from academic staff.
There is a need for reassurance that assessment practices are adequate
and relevant. In particular, it has been documented that mentors have
fears about failing students (Ilott, 1997; Hopkins, 2000), and so avoid
confronting issues. This is of grave concern in a practice-based profession where, if we are to maintain self-regulation, the assessment of a
student's clinical practice should be documented and defensible (Searle,

2000). Mentors require support from lecturers regarding assessment, particularly when addressing difficult issues with students. Effective support from lecturers can increase the mentor's confidence in their abilities and this in turn can enhance the student's experience.

Although there is great potential for the link lecturer role to have an impact on practice-based learning, because of difficulties in fulfilling the full remit of the role, there have been many attempts to instigate alternative models.

Lecturer practitioner (LP) roles

Initially after the phasing out of the clinical lecturer role in the mid-1980s, various models for joint appointments (King's Fund, 1984), and lecturer practitioners (Fitzgerald, 1989) were instigated on a trial basis in some areas throughout the UK. These initiatives met with limited success unless fully endorsed by successful partnerships with practice units and unless the overall philosophy of the curriculum content, structure and organization supported the continued development of the role (Lathlean, 1995). The enthusiasm and hard work of the particular incumbents of these innovative roles was a major factor in their success. There is evidence that ideas for the development of new models for the role of the lecturer in practice continued into the 1990s. Of these new models, the lecturer practitioner (LP) continues to dominate in terms of numbers and scope.

Following its early development in Oxford (Lathlean, 1995), the LP model continues to be a viable option for supporting students in practice (Fairbrother and Ford, 1996; Hollingworth, 1997; Graham *et al.*, 2001). There has been a growth in the number of appointments to the LP role, with reinterpretations and increasing variability in how the role is implemented (Williamson and Webb, 2001). Although work has been done to describe the scope and function of the role, to date its outcome effectiveness has not been evaluated.

All stakeholders, including students, practitioners and education staff, have responded positively to the LP role. However, it has been noted that the majority of appointments to the role have a focus in supporting qualified staff who are completing post-registration educational programmes (Day *et al.*, 1998). Similar to the clinical teacher role in the past, although the LP role is satisfying for individual teachers, some difficulties have been highlighted, especially in relation to dealing with the competing demands of a dual post and in establishing a career pathway.

In the Jones (1996) and Fairbrother and Ford (1996) studies, respondents highlighted that there were no career paths as they did not 'belong' to either education or service.

The LP posts have been established on an *ad hoc* basis and in response to local needs. Funding restraints are the main reason for not instigating these posts. Trusts rather than the universities predominantly hold contracts of employment, though funding is shared by both types of institution (Andrewes, 2001; Hollingworth, 1997).

The main focus for the continuing establishment of LP posts arises from the perceived benefits to students, practitioners and the lecturers. These benefits include:

• promoting effective collaboration between education and service;
• advancing research-based practice;
• developing nursing practice;
• facilitating the application of theory to practice;
• lecturing from a clinically credible base.

While post-registration courses in nursing continue to be well supported through the growth of LP posts, it has been recognized that students completing pre-registration programmes are not adequately supported through the current role of the lecturer in practice (Day *et al.*, 1998;. UKCC 1999; DOH, 1999).

The practice teacher/educator

Emphasis within recent policy documents (DOH, 1999; 2000) is on ensuring a high quality of practice teaching, with a clear remit that those with recent practice experience should undertake the role of practice teacher/educator. Formalizing the mentorship role and allowing time out for practitioners to develop their clinical teaching skills is necessary for providing high-quality support for students in practice environments (UKCC, 2000). As part of a policy re-emphasis on practice education, new documents from both the UKCC (2000) and the DOH/ENB (2001a) have re-emphasized quality outcome standards for mentors, practice educators and lecturers on nursing, midwifery and health visiting.

In identifying the differences between a lecturer and a practice educator, DOH/ENB (2001a) indicates that the practice educator makes a significant contribution to education in the practice setting. A practice educator is expected to:

- coordinate student experiences;
- oversee assessments of practice learning;
- provide support and guidance for mentors;
- identify the professional development needs of the team and ensure they are met;
- lead the development of practice (DOH/ENB, 2001)

The above role functions represent a large remit for the practice educator role. It is interesting to note that actual 'clinical teaching' is not included in the role descriptors, as the primary responsibility for practice teaching still rests with the practitioner as mentor. It could be argued that one of the ways practice educators can provide guidance for mentors is through role modelling clinical/practice teaching. Working directly with the student/mentor dyad in taking a patient case load can be a very effective way of supporting both student and mentor.

In providing a list of programme outcomes for the development of practice educators and practice education, the UKCC (2000) emphasizess knowledge and skills related to:

- communication
- facilitation of practice learning
- assessment
- role modelling
- creating a learning environment
- practice development
- research appraisal and evaluation.

Any training course or work-based learning approach to developing practice educators would need to address the fostering of this knowledge and these skills. It is assumed that, as a prerequisite, the practice educators will work in their areas of practice expertise and will remain grounded within that area. Good-quality teaching in whatever context develops with experience, work, time, self-reflection and supportive mentoring.

It should be recognized that the most significant contribution to developing skills in practice teaching are the key personal skills of the individual educator. Practice teaching is unlike traditional classroom teaching. It is unpredictable, emotional, seldom static and creates unique challenges for the individual teacher (White and Ewan, 1991; Karuhije 1997; Ludwick *et al.*, 1998). There are potential problems in dealing with the time-consuming nature of clinical teaching. These include safety concerns and the need for flexibility and adaptability of approach to the rapidly changing demands of the practice area and the learning needs of the individual student. The re-emergence of specialist modules within teacher preparation programmes that will specifically address the challenges of practice-based teaching is a welcome development for the future (DOH/ENB, 2001a).

Models for the future

Planned increases in the numbers of trained healthcare professionals have highlighted the need for expansion in the number and quality of placement areas (DOH, 2000a). New and stronger partnerships between service providers and HEIs need to be created to address the problem.

Partnership posts – the bournemouth model of collaborative development

The creation of new education management posts within NHS Trusts, such as the 'Practice Placement Facilitator' or a 'Lead Nurse for Clinical Education', has shifted the focal base for the development of practice learning environments back to the health service providers. The need for an accountable individual who is based in practice and who has a remit to develop the learning environment for all healthcare professionals has been recognized (DOH/ENB, 2001a). Currently the creation of 'new' roles in practice teaching that are primarily based within the practice areas echoes the past role of clinical teachers. In contrast to the clinical teacher posts of the 1970s/80s, these new posts of 'practice teacher/educator' are predominantly managed by NHS Trusts as opposed to the HEIs. However, incumbents of these roles will work in strong partnership with the local education provider.

Service providers are also undertaking the management of the infrastructure support for practice-based education. Through proposals to create within NHS Trusts senior management posts in clinical education coordination, the specific support required at a local level will be recognized.

The Bournemouth model of collaborative development (Dorset and South Wiltshire Education Purchasing Consortium, 2001) is a good example of a partnership initiative especially designed to support pre-registration nursing students in practice placements. New posts at senior nursing management level (assistant directors of nursing) with the title of

Co-ordinator of Clinical Education have been instigated in all the major acute NHS Trusts providing placements for student nurses. Specialist senior posts to support students from the branches of nursing where practice placements are predominantly within primary care (Mental Health, Leaning Disabilities, Child Health) have been based within the university (see Figure 8.1).

Each of these NHS senior post-holders, in partnership with the local HEI, deals with issues such as:

- developing and auditing of practice learning environments in line with Quality Assurance Agency (QAA, 2001) requirements;
- preparing and initiating new areas for practice learning;
- monitoring and adjusting practice placements in response to local service pressures and changes;
- maintaining an active register of mentors/assessors;
- managing a locally based team of practice teachers/educators, LPs and link lecturers.

At local Trust level, these senior managers are active and prominent at a strategic level in promoting a quality learning environment for all NHS professionals, in developing an education strategy for the Trust, and being active in providing an infrastructure to monitor and measure continuous professional development (CPD) needs of all staff. The post-holder, in certain Trusts that provide an infrastructure of support for National Vocational Qualifications (NVQs) for their healthcare support workers, will manage the NVQ facilitator's team. The coordinator is also expected to recognize and promote any local Trust opportunities for multiprofessional learning.

Teams of practice educators (PEs) are being appointed who have specific clinical expertise and skills, and commitment to teaching and facilitating students in the practice environment. Under the management and leadership of the coordinators of clinical education, these practice educators are locality based and provide full-time support to students and mentors in an allocated number of wards/units/areas. An example is one PE in a full-time post who provides education support for five elderly care/rehabilitation wards. The educator has extensive experience and degree-level education in elderly care with a commitment to the development of elderly care nursing. Individual Trusts have appointed PEs in Surgery, Orthopaedics, Medicine and Elderly Care. Primary Care Trusts will have a PE who will focus on facilitating practice learning support

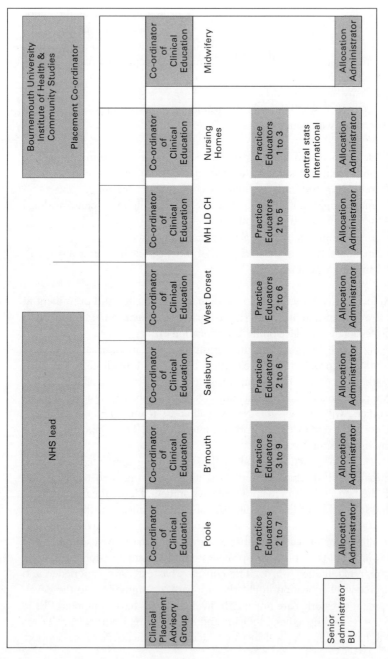

Figure 8.1 Bournemouth model of collaborative development

138

across the community teams, providing adult patient/client care within the locality.

Practice educators already have teaching qualifications obtained through completion of the ENB 998 or equivalent courses. Their knowledge and skills will be developed further through completing a postgraduate diploma in Education to include an emphasis on undertaking the Practice Educator Programme as outlined by the UKCC (UKCC, 2000).

Growth in the number of PE posts will take place within a three-year time frame. These new partnership posts, funded through a local education confederation and currently being instigated, need ongoing evaluation of their effectiveness in providing for quality practice-based learning. An infrastructure of support has been set up for the team of coordinators of clinical education and the practice educators themselves. Practice Placement Education Steering and Operational Groups have been established by the HEI. Evaluation of the initiative is being managed through Bournemouth University's Education Research Unit.

The Bournemouth model described above needed vision and commitment by the University senior education and the local NHS Trusts partnership team. Considerable financial resources were needed to set up the initiative, and the continuing support of the local education consortium/confederation is essential to maintain this development in the future.

Practice learning teams – the Nottingham model

Partnership developments also recognize the need for variety and flexibility to address local educational needs. The various roles of link lecturers, lecturer practitioners, practice teacher/educators and mentors can be harnessed to provide an integrated team approach for a group of practice learning areas through the instigation of a 'practice learning team'.

Traditionally, practice links have been viewed as educationalists providing support/liaison to placement areas, with advice being given on educational matters. However, all organizations and professions need to share the responsibility of supporting and educating the next generation of healthcare professionals (DOH/ENB, 2001). There is a need for collaborative working, with a change of climate to enable true working in partnership (Williamson and Webb, 2001). The historical view of lecturers providing support for practice may have actually contributed, to some degree, to the 'them and us' approach to the education of student nurses. An achievable goal, for the foreseeable future, is not for a university lecturer to take on a clinical teaching role, but rather for educationalists to help practitioners facilitate learning and provide adequate support for the learning environment that will enhance practice learning for students (MacNeil, 1997).

In Nottingham, it was recognized that a new system of support needed to be developed. The education team acknowledged that while there were pockets of excellence in terms of supporting practice learning, the link lecturer system was not uniformly effective, not consistent across all placement areas, and expectations of the role were unclear for all stakeholders (Day *et al.*, 1998). In addition, a general lack of guidance for and monitoring and management of the lecturer's practice role tended to imply little role value. This lack of value appears to be reinforced when there is little or no formal preparation for the practice role within current teaching courses. Varied interpretations of the role led to considerable difficulty in determining its purpose, with this lack of clarity leading to difficulty in establishing criteria to evaluate effectiveness.

In reviewing these findings, it was decided to hold three one-day workshops inviting lecturers, practitioners, service managers and students. The purpose of the workshops was to review where we were in terms of practice support, where we would like to be and how we were going to get there.

Practitioners, teachers and students who attended the workshops found that:

- the current system of allocating link lecturers to provide educational support to practice areas was not uniformly effective;
- the methods lecturers use to maintain and provide links are not consistent across all placement areas;
- expectations of the link lecturer role is unclear to teaching staff, practice staff and students;
- it is difficult to find replacements when link lecturers leave the organization. This results in some practice areas being left without an allocated educational link person.

These findings are similar to those outlined from a national study by Day *et al.* (1998). The workshops therefore reinforced current research findings, and the outcome was that more effective support for practice learning was necessary. A team approach was the favoured method of achieving this, with lecturers and practitioners working in partnership. At the same time, Nottingham was chosen as a 'Making a Difference' curriculum demonstration site, and this development offered further impetus in terms of reformulating the practice support systems in place.

The Nottingham School of Nursing is a large school covering both rural and urban areas over three counties. There are 200 lecturers to support 2400 placement areas. The logistical challenges in providing support for this number of placements are tremendous. A consultation exercise was undertaken involving staff at all levels: teaching staff, practitioners, trust managers and members of the Education Confederation. Commitment was required from all parties to ensure that the teams would be successful in helping to improve the current situation.

The constitution of practice learning teams (PLTs)

Membership of the practice learning teams is likely to differ depending on the unit/directorate and/or group of placements involved. However, it was envisaged that the teams would consist of a combination of School of Nursing and practice staff. For example, in Health Services for Elderly Care in one NHS Trust, a team made up of six lecturers and 16 practitioners covers the learning needs of approximately fifty students on 16 placement areas.

All lecturers with a responsibility for teaching and supporting pre- and post-registration students were expected to participate in at least one practice learning team. Practitioner representatives form part of each team, to provide advice and support to the team on current practice issues. Each team elects an individual to act as the team leader/coordinator. Team roles include support and advice to assessors on learning and teaching matters, provision of support for students in practice, updating staff on curriculum matters and providing support to practice managers. A member of the team, ideally the team leader, will attend unit/directorate meetings in order to generate shared discussions regarding educational matters. In the smaller branches of nursing, for examples learning disabilities, teachers from other branches may form part of the learning disability team to assist with assessor and student support only.

The functions of the PLTs are as follows:

- strengthening the partnerships between practice and education by providing a tangible presence;

- developing, facilitating and supporting students' practice-based learning;
- providing a forum for sharing 'good practice' and the exchange of information;
- developing initiatives that enhance practice-based learning;
- participating in the update of assessors;
- acting as a resource for the professional development of practice staff;
- providing feedback to practice staff about students' evaluation of their placement experience;
- contributing to the School of Nursing educational audit process.

Apart from general aims developed centrally, the teams, once established, were encouraged to develop team roles according to their local needs and wants. Whilst it could be argued that this could lead to inconsistency between teams, it was seen to be important for team members to have a sense of ownership of their team, with the autonomy to develop new initiatives in relation to practice learning. It is interesting to note that teams have evolved similar models to operationalize the system, but also new ideas generated through individual teams have been shared with all teams as well as problems encountered and how they have been overcome.

We have had some difficulties. Some teams are working more effectively than others. However, the initiative is still in its infancy. Currently we have 46 teams established across the five sites of the School. Learning Disabilities, Mental Health and the Child Branches have a cross-school organizer for the teams, whereas for the Adult Branch someone is designated to organize the teams at each of the five sites in the School. The challenge is to support and encourage the less effective teams in their development, and this will be monitored through the management structures in place for teams.

Support for mentors who facilitate learning in practice is an issue of concern. Through the PLTs, the mentoring updating and support they provide can concentrate on local issues and needs, with both teachers and practitioners sharing the responsibility for the updating of mentors and facilitating and monitoring learning.

The teams also give teaching staff support for the practice aspect of their role, together with some preparation for the role. Education and practice are developing their philosophy regarding practice education as well as identifying the learning opportunities available for differing levels of students within an area. In doing this we are beginning to develop some sort of yardstick by which a student's progress and level of achievement can be measured. This has the advantage of helping to increase consistency within the mentoring and assessing roles.

PLTs are increasingly becoming involved in practice-based learning (PBL). This is theory time on the course that is devoted to preparing students for their placement experience, developing their skills and knowledge, and helping them to reflect on their experiences. The involvement of PLT members in practice-based learning helps to reflect the value placed upon practice experience. Teaching staff have the educational expertise and practitioners have current nursing practice expertise. In working together, using the expertise of different members of the team, we are learning from each other, ensuring that the methods used for learning are effective and the knowledge and skills gained by students are appropriate for today's practice. The curriculum has the potential to become more dynamic as the PLTs are more able to respond quickly to changes within practice, and to student needs.

Etablishing a team approach between practitioners and lecturers has given an opportunity for both parties to appreciate the difficulties inherent in each other's roles. A team approach allows the participants to identify priorities within the areas they focus upon, with shared responsibility and ideas potentially leading to innovative approaches to practice learning. A team approach is also developmental for lecturers and practitioners: practitioners can develop their educational role and lecturers can develop their practice roles.

Research by Day *et al.* (1998) highlighted the need for a managed system to support the practice curriculum. A managed structure is necessary to assist a proactive approach to practice learning, helping to ensure demarcated time for all parties, facilitating some consistency regarding practice support, and helping to establish support for those new to the lecturer's and mentor's role. More importantly, it enables the monitoring and evaluation of the initiative as a whole.

The PLTs are a managed system. There is a school coordinator for the initiative who reports to the Practice Development Committee, which is an executive group whose remit is the strategic development of practice. The school coordinator of the PLTs has the responsibility for overseeing the implementation and development of the teams, working in close conjunction with the clinical placement development facilitators, who are Trust employees. Other responsibilities of the school coordinator include the sharing of examples of best practice as well as problems encountered and how these are being managed by individual teams.

The coordinator also reports formally on a monthly basis to the Practice Development Commitee, with an annual report of achievement of objectives and action plans identified for the next year.

The managed system allows a two-way communication and encourages the communication of successes, new initiatives and difficulties encountered. It also enables a formal forum for issues to be discussed and plans for development of such an important initiative.

Although formal evaluations have yet to be undertaken, there has been tremendous enthusiasm for the team approach. Practitioner members in particular have welcomed the opportunity to participate in the shaping of teams, with some teams being led by a practitioner. This helps to reinforce the commitment we have to working in true partnership. Sharing the processes involved to date is a priority, with conference presentations as a first step to disseminating information about the PLTs (Aston and Chapple, 2001).

International comparisons

Nurse education in the USA, Canada and Australia has been integrated into the higher education sector for considerably longer than in the UK. Shifting from the traditional apprenticeship system of education, as in the UK, means that the student becomes supernumerary while undertaking their clinical experiences. In all of these countries the responsibility for practice education was devolved to the university sector. Clinical educators in one form or another are employed to supervise the learning needs of students in the practice setting. Employing clinical educators is an expensive option for the HE sector, and many models have evolved to provide quality practice teaching in a cost-effective way (Melander and Roberts, 1994; Greenwood and Winifreyda, 1995; Ferguson, 1996; Nordgren *et al.*, 1998).

Recent shifts in thinking appear to favour a move towards the more active involvement of practitioners in taking responsibility for student learning in the USA. However, there are rewards and bargaining systems in place so that practitioners who partner students will be given associate lecturing roles (Nordgen *et al.*, 1998).

In Australia, the professional requirement for a set number of hours in practice for registration is also being achieved though the instigation of extensive facilities for clinical laboratory sessions on campus (Mallik, 1995). This allows students to develop psychomotor clinical skills in a safe environment where they are supervised and tested by lecturing staff.

In the UK, there is evidence of the reinstatement of clinical learning laboratories as a viable system for teaching clinical skills in the UK (Nichol and Glen, 1999). Involvement in practice education, both in the skills laboratory in the university and in the practice area, should be a viable option for lecturers and practice educators.

Conclusion

Growing criticism of the lack of 'fitness for practice' of registered nurses educated through the 'new' diploma level courses instigated in the UK in the late 1980s led to the recommendations in *Fitness for Practice* (UKCC, 1999). These recommendations called for a re-evaluation of the provision of practice education, with equal emphasis on the quality of educational support offered to learners in practice areas and in the classroom.

A culture of 'clinical education by default' (Edmond, 2001) was seen to devalue the importance of learning in practice, with the achievement of academic award being the higher priority for academic institutions. It was hoped that, once registered, the newly qualified staff nurse would 'pick up' the skills required to provide care and make clinical decisions. A 'cycle of deprivation' was set up in which in order to make up for the deficit in 'fitness for practice' at registration, the support of newly qualified staff nurses in their transition period became part of a portfolio of continuous professional development supplied by their employers (Gerrish, 2000; McClean and Smith, 2000; Mallik and Bennett, 2001; Mallik and Toulson, 2002).

A concerted effort is now being made to turn the recommendations of *Fitness for Practice* (UKCC, 1999) into reality. With the refocusing of attention on developing constructive partnerships between service providers of healthcare and the HEIs, a number of different innovative approaches are being instigated and evaluated. As stated in recommendation 25 (UKCC, 1999, p. 48),

> recognising that no one individual can provide for the full range of expertise required by students, service providers and HEIs should work together to develop diverse teams of practice and academic staff who will offer students expertise in practice, management, assessment, mentoring and research.

The Nottingham model of instigating practice learning teams is one way forward. It provides for more effective use of current resources through genuine partnership working and is relatively cost neutral. Investing in and developing a team of practice educators, organized and managed by a senior NHS service manager (Bournemouth model) is another way forward. However, it is important to recognize the local nature of these innovations.

Continuation of the process of contracting with educational consortia for the provision of education for health service professionals means that the cost of providing practice learning support for nurses, midwives and health visitors is in a competitive position with other demands on education funding. Providing structured support for clinical education is expensive. Although national strategy documents support quality education in practice (DOH/ENB, 2001), because of diminishing funding and increased demands, developments may continue to be *ad hoc* and subject to local action by key visionary stakeholders. Providing a nursing workforce that is 'fit for practice' in the future demands a fight for the vision of structured support for quality practice learning now. The lecturer/practice educator must continue to play a key supportive role in practice learning.

References

Andrewes, C (2001) Clinical Academic Pathways – A Collaborative Model, *National LP Forum Newsletter*, Spring 2001, London: Foundation of Nursing Studies.

Aston, E (2000) Assessing students in clinical practice. Unpublished MSc dissertation, Nottingham, The University of Nottingham.

Aston, E and Chapple, M (2001) Practice Learning Teams: A way of improving the quality of student learning in practice. Unpublished Paper, Nurse Education Today Conference, September 2001, Durham, UK.

Aston, E, Mallik, M, Day, C and Fraser, D (2000) An exploration of the teacher/lecturer in practice – findings from a case study in adult nursing, *Nurse Education Today*, **17**(3), 175–82.

Clifford, C (1993) The clinical role of the nurse teacher in the UK, *Journal of Advanced Nursing*, **18**(2), 218–19.

Collins, A, Brown, J S, Newman, S E (1989) Cognitive Apprenticeship: teaching the crafts of reading writing and mathematics. In Resnick, L B (ed.), *Knowing, Learning and Instruction: Essays in honor of Robert Glaser*. Hillsdale, NJ: Erlbaum, pp. 453–94.

Day, C, Fraser, D and Mallik, M (1998) *The role of the nurse teacher/lecturer in practice. Researching Professional Education No 8*. London: ENB.

Department of Health (1999) *Making a Difference: Strengthening the nursing, midwifery and health visiting contribution to health and health care*. London: DOH.

Department of Health (2000) Consultative Document, *A Health Service for all Talents: Developing the NHS workforce*. London: DOH.

Department of Health (2000a) *The NHS Plan: A plan for investment, a plan for reform.* London: DOH.

Department of Health/English National Board (2001) *Placements in Focus: Guidance for Education in Practice for Health Care Professionals.* London: DOH/ENB.

Department of Health/English National Board (2001a) *Preparation of Mentors and Teachers: A new framework of guidance.* London, DOH/ENB.

Dorset and South Wiltshire Education Purchasing Consortium (2001) Practice Teaching Framework to support the new Pre-Registration Nursing Curriculum for Adult and Child Branch (unpublished proposal). Bournemouth: DSWEPC.

Duffy K (2000) The nurse lecturer's role in mentoring the mentors, *Nursing Standard*, **15**(6) 35–8.

Edmond, C B (2001) A new paradigm for practice education, *Nurse Education Today*, **21**, 251–59.

English National Board (1985) *Professional Education/Training Courses: Consultation paper.* London: ENB.

English National Board (1989) *Preparation of Teachers, Practitioner Teachers, Mentors and Supervisors in the context of P2000.* London: ENB.

English National Board (1995) *Regulations and guidelines for the approval of Education Institutions and Programmes.* London: ENB.

English National Board (1997) *Standards for the approval of HEIs and Programes.* London, ENB.

Eraut, M (1999) *Developing Professional Knowledge and Competence*, 4th edn. London,: Farmer Press.

Fairbrother, P and Ford, S (1996) *Mapping the Territory: Lecturer-Practitioners in Trent Region.* Sheffield: Postgraduate and Research Centre, University of Sheffield.

Ferguson D (1996) The lived experience of Clinical Educators, *Journal of Advanced Nursing*, **23**(4), 835–41.

Fitzgerald, M (1989) Lecturer Practitioner: Action Researcher. Unpublished MN thesis, Cardiff, University of Wales.

Fretwell, J E (1982) *Ward teaching and Learning.* London: RCN.

Gerrish, C (2000) Still fumbling along? A comparative study of the newly qualified nurse's perception of the transition from student to qualified nurse. *Journal of Advanced Nursing*, **32**(2), 473–80.

Graham, I, Andrewes, C and Galvin, K (2001) Bournemouth's new initiative: A Clinical University. *National Lecturer Practitioner Forum Newsletter*, Winter. London: Foundation of Nursing Studies.

Greenwood, J and Winifreyda, A (1995) Two strategies for promotong clinical competence in pre-registration nursing students, *Nurse Education Today*, **15**(3), 184–89.

Hancock, P (1999) Reflective practice – using a learning journal, *Nursing Standard*, **13**(7),37–40.

Hollingworth, S (1997) *Lecturer Practitioner Roles in England (Executive summary Report)*. London: DOH.

Hopkins S (2000) *The Student Experience at the Central Sheffield University Hospitals*, The Central Sheffield University Hospitals.

Ilott, I (1997) Feelings and failings in professional training: the assessor's dilemma. *Assessment and Evaluation in Higher Education*, **22**(3), 162–7.

Jones, H M (1996) Introducing a lecturer-practitioner: the management perspective, *Journal of Nursing Management*, **4**, 337–45.

Karuhjie, H F (1997) Classroom and clinical teaching in nursing: Delineating differences, *Nursing Forum*, **32**(2), 5–12.

King's Fund (1984) *Joint Clinical–Teaching Appointments in Nursing*. London: King Edward's Hospital Fund for London.

Kirkwood L (1979) The Clinical Teacher, *Nursing Times (Occasional Paper)*, **75**(12), 49–51.

Lathlean, J (1995) *The implementation and development of lecturer-practitioner roles in nursing*. Oxford: Ashdale Press.

Ludwick, R, Dieckman, B C, Herdtner, S, Dugan, M and Roche, M (1998) Documenting the scholarship of clinical teaching through peer review, *Nurse Educator*, **23**(6), 17–20.

Luker, K, Carlisle, C and Kirk, S (1995) *The evolving role of the nurse teacher in the light of educational reforms*. London: ENB.

McClean, J and Smith, M (2000) *The Effectiveness of a Competency-Based Preceptor programme for Newly Qualified and Newly Employed Staff Nurses. Final Report. Edinburgh:* National Board for Scotland.

MacNeil,M (1997) From nurse to teacher: recognising a status passage, *Journal of Advanced Nursing*, **25**(3), 634–42.

Mallik, M (1995) *Developing Reflective Practitioners: the Role of the Nurse Educator*. London: Report to the Florence Nightingale Foundation

Mallik, M and Bennett C (2001) The Supervised Post Diploma Development Year Project. Unpublished Final Report. London: Royal Free Hampstead (NHS) Trust and Middlesex University.

Mallik, M and Toulson, A (2002) The Preceptorship Degree Programme – A Review. Unpublished Report. Salisbury Health Care Trust and Bournemouth University.

Martin, L (1989) *Clinical Education in Perspective*. London: Royal College of Nursing.

Melander, S and Roberts, C (1994) Clinical Teaching Associate Model: Creating effective BSN student/faculty/staff nurse triads, *Journal of Nurse Education*, **33**(9), 422–5.

Ministry of Health (1966) *Report of the Committee on Senior Nursing Structure (The Salmon Report)*. London: HMSO.

Neary, M (1999) Preparing assessors for continuous assessment, *Nursing Standard*, **13**(18), 41–7.

Nichol, M and Glen, S (1999) *Clinical Skills in Nursing – The return of the practical room?* Basingstoke: Macmillan – now Palgrave Macmillan.

Nordgren, J, Richardson, S J and Laurella, V B (1998) A Collaborative Preceptor Model for Clinical Teaching of Beginning Nursing Students, *Nurse Educator*, **23**(3), 27–32.

Ogier, M E (1982) *An Ideal Sister?* London: Royal College of Nursing.

Orton, H D (1981) *Ward Learning Climate*. London: RCN.

Phillips, T, Schostak, J, Bedford, H and Robinson, J (1994) *Education, Dialogue and Assessment: creating partnerships for improving practice – A report based on assessing competencies in nursing and midwifery education (the ACE report)*. Researching Professional Education Series No. 1. London: ENB.

Quality Assurance Agency for Higher Education (2001) *Code of Practice for the Assurance of Academic Quality and Standards in H.E.: Placement Learning.* http://www.qaa.ac.uk/public/cop/copplacement/appendix2.htm

Quality Support Centre (1995a) *Developing Student's Subject Knowledge in the Workplace: Annotated bibliography*. London, Open University and DfEE.

Quality Support Centre (1995b) *Developing Students' Subject Knowledge in the Workplace; Guidelines for good practice in supporting students in the workplace*. London: Open University and DfEE.

Quality Support Centre (1995c*) Developing Students' Subject Knowledge in the Workplace; Signpost for Staff Development (1): Link Tutors*. London, Open University & DfEE.

Quality Support Centre (1995d) *Developing Student's Subject Knowledge in the Workplace: Signpost for Staff Development (2): Workplace Mentors*. London: Open University and DfEE.

Quality Support Centre (1995e*) Developing Students' Subject Knowledge in the Workplace: Signpost for Staff Development (3): Student Peer Support*. London: Open University and DfEE.

Robertson, C M (1987) *A very special form of Teaching*. London: Royal College of Nursing.

Searle, J (2000) Defining competency – the role of standard setting, *Medical Education*, **34**(5), 363–6.

Smith, A (1998), Learning about reflection, *Journal of Advanced Nursing*, **28**(4), 891–8.

Taylor, L K and Dean Care, W (1999) Nurse Education as Cognitive Apprenticeship: A framework for clinical education, *Nurse Educator*, **24**(4), 31–6.

UKCC (1999), *Fitness for Practice* – The UKCC Commission for Nursing and Midwifery Education chaired by Sir Leonard Peach. London: UKCC.

UKCC (2000), *Standards for the Preparation of Teachers of Nursing, Midwifery and Health Visiting*. London: UKCC.

Watson, H E and Harris, B (1999) *Supporting Students in Practice Placements in Scotland – an NBS commissioned Study*: Glasgow, Glasgow Caledonian University.

White, E, Davies, S, Twinn, S and Riley E (1993) *A detailed study of the relationship between teaching, support, supervision and role modelling for students in clinical areas within the context of P2000 courses.* London: ENB.

White, R and Ewan, C (1991) *Clinical Teaching in Nursing.* London: Chapman & Hall.

Williamson, G R and Webb, C (2001) Supporting students in practice, *Journal of Clinical Nursing*, **10**(2), 284–92.

9

Towards a New Paradigm for Practice Education

Sally Glen

Introduction

The previous chapters have demonstrated that the problems associated with a culture of clinical education by default (unavailability of physical and human resources and few collaborative structures, see Chapter 1) have, since the late 1990s, been defined and redefined. It is now time to move on. This will require the following: new models of partnership between educators and practising professionals; the development of academic/practice career pathways; a new model of practice education; and the generation of research-based evidence and scholarship that informs policy development and best practice.

New models of partnership

The shift of nursing to higher education in the late 1980s and early 1990s resulted in the enhancement of educational standards and contributed to the professionalization of nursing (see Chapter 3). Using research into nurse education published in the mid-1990s, Corbett (1998) writes about how nurse education and service delivery were uncoupled. Breckenridge (2002), as an academic doctor, similarly notes concern over many years about the problems arising at the interface between higher education and the NHS. This is therefore not only a nursing issue. As each of the previous chapters has demonstrated, since the late 1990s, there has been increasing recognition of appropriate sharing of responsibility for students' practice learning between HEIs and service providers (see Chapter 1).

Partnership: HEIs and service providers

The notion of partnership between service providers and HEIs is, of course, not new (see Chapter 1). For example, the UKCC document *A Statement of Strategic Intent* (UKCC, 1994) emphasized the need for collaboration at every level in the provision of both pre- and post-registration nurse education. This document argued that such partnerships should place the students at the centre of the learning experience within a framework that is practice led, research based and employment focused. This was re-emphasized in *Making a Difference* (DOH, 1999) and *Fitness for Practice* (UKCC, 1999) (see Chapter 3). Recommendation 25 (p. 48) states that:

> Recognising that no one individual can provide the full range of expertise required by students, service providers and HEI's should work together to develop diverse teams of practice and academic staff who will offer students expertise in practice, management, assessment and mentoring and research.

Following recommendations arising from *Fitness for Practice* and *Making a Difference*, there has been a greater focus on developing partnerships between service providers and HEIs (Glen, 2000). The NHS review of workforce planning (DOH, 2000a), *The NHS Plan* (DOH, 2000b), *Working Together, Learning Together* (DOH, 2001a), the National Audit Office Report (2001) and the Royal College of Nursing (2002) all reinforce the expectation that all health and social care organizations should play a part in working closely with higher education and professional and statutory bodies to expand placement capacity and provide an environment that facilitates learning. The Department of Health and the Higher Education Funding Council for England (2000a) announced a *Statement of Strategic Alliance for Health and Social Care*. Practice placements are referred to in this document (p. 4) as a 'key area of commitment' and thus:

> The DOH and HEFCE are commited to working together to ensure the provision of sufficient and appropriate practice placements to a wide range of NHS trusts, primary care, wider health care sector and social care settings.

The wider use of funding in support of placements has been examined as part of the review of the Multi-Professional Education and Training Levy (MPET). The Department of Health (2002b) in its document suggests that overtime placement support should be redirected to support all healthcare students training in the NHS (not just medical students as it is presently). It states (p. 3): Placement funding should support teaching activity, common learning during clinical placements, and more multidisciplinary use of clinical teaching facilities.' In essence, it recommends funding for dedicated time in education for practice staff and dedicated time in practice for lecturers to support interprofessional education.

Each of the chapters in this book has reinforced the premise that an effective working relationship between HEIs and service-based organizations is fundamental to the development of practice placements.

Partnership: across HEIs and service organizations

The management of placements across organizations can prove beneficial in improving their quality and capacity. A group is often formed to map existing and potential placements and to discuss with HEIs the number of students requiring placements (NHS Executive, 2000). Such a group can also consider a variety of placement models to maximize quality and capacity. For example, applying a hospital placement model to primary and community care settings generally does not work. The organizational structure within hospitals is generally hierarchical by profession. This does not reflect structures within the community. The small multiprofessional team nature of primary and community care requires a different approach.

One suggested way forward is to establish links between HEIs, service organizations and Workforce Development Confederations (WDCs) to determine the current situation regarding the range of practice placements across professions. The process might involve developing:

- a managed approach to identifying, developing and monitoring placement learning opportunities,
- new learning opportunities to meet contemporary practice in accordance with both locally and nationally determined standards,
- common learning outcomes in practice,
- one educational audit tool and assessment tools,
- common placement supervision/teachers,

- partnerships across professions,
- common student expectations.

Examples of good practice developed across institutions also include WDC-wide 'Practice Experience Units', which may be 'actual' or 'virtual', to share placements across all Trusts and universities linked to the WDC. In order to increase placement capacity and capability, and the spend on skills development, the provision of a placement unit alongside e-learning facilities and integrated learning resources as supportive of, and complementary to, placement learning, an integrated healthcare learning network is one possible way forward.

The concept of such a network is based on the premise that professional knowledge, skills and attitudes are no longer bound by time and place, but can occur at any time. Over time an integrated healthcare learning network could consist of the components shown in Figure 9.1.

The principal aims are to:

- optimize the provision and facilitate the effective utilization of educational resources (in particular IT, library, media resources and placements),
- promote interprofessional education and practice through the utilization of a range of innovative learning and teaching strategies (in particular e-based learning),
- increase local placement capacity and quality and implement a viable mechanism for providing interprofessional practice experience,
- increase partnership working between universities, local Acute Trusts, Primary Care Trusts and local social and voluntary agencies.

A major challenge is to accommodate increasing numbers of healthcare students without imposing unnecessary burdens on service staff or compromising service delivery.

Partnership: across professions

Interprofessional education has undoubtedly been given increasing momentum as a result of the *NHS Plan* (DOH, 2000b); other key documents include:

- *A Health Service of All The Talents: Developing The NHS Workforce* (DOH, 2000a) (blurring of professional boundaries)

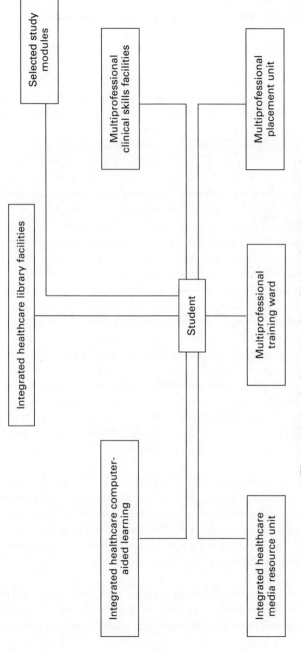

Figure 9.1 An integrated healthcare learning network

- *Working Together, Learning Together: A Framework for Lifelong Learning in the NHS* (DOH, 2001a) (changing roles and workforce design)
- *Shifting the Balance* (DOH, 2001b) (cross-sector and cross-agency working)

All the above also reinforce the expectation that all health and social care organizations should play a part in working together with HEIs to provide an environment that facilitates interprofessional education, and expands placement quality and capacity.

Research into the effects of interprofessional education is beginning to identify a favourable range of outcomes associated with this activity (see Chapter 7). As noted in Chapter 7, these include enhancing teamwork skills and improving knowledge of different professional roles (Barr, 2001). However, there has been no attempt to systematically investigate the longer-term impact of interprofessional education. Therefore there is uncertainty about its impact on clients and patients. In an attempt to address this shortfall, two systematic reviews of the effectiveness of interprofessional education have been undertaken.

A 'Cochrane Review' focused on only those studies that employ one of three research designs (randomized controlled trials; controlled before-and-after studies, and interrupted time-series studies). In addition, this review focused on two types of outcome: changes in professional practice and/or changes in the care delivered to clients/patients. It found no studies that met these criteria (Zwarenstein *et al.*, 1999). In order to understand the wider effects of interprofessional education (using a broader range of methods), a second review has been undertaken (Koppel *et al.* 2001). The aim of this review is to be as robust as the first, but less constrained in terms of methodology and outcome. Initial findings from a search of 'Medline' suggest:

- Work-based interprofessional education that has a duration over two weeks tends to report a positive impact on clients and patients (for example, reducing length of stays, client/patient satisfaction).
- Work-based interprofessional education appears to have more impact on clients and patients in acute care settings rather than chronic care settings.

Preliminary evaluation therefore suggests that work-based interprofessional education is much more likely than university-based education to positively affect clients and patients (Cable, 2000). Learning and exposure to good role models in placements has of course long been recognized as more influential than learning and role models within educational institutions (see Chapter 1). *Fitness for Practice* (UKCC, 1999, Recommendation 32, p. 52) recommends:

- Purchasers of education include interprofessional teaching and learning as a criterion for evaluating the quality of education.
- The development of shared use of learning resources and technology in practice placements.

Tope (1996) also argues that learning about interprofessional working is best achieved when students interact in 'real-life' situations. It is generally accepted that adult learning is more likely to be effective if it is interactive and problem-case or task focused. Practice placements, therefore, provide an ideal setting for students to develop and practise interprofessional collaboration skills, especially when the placements are in service settings, where different professions are involved in patient care. However, traditionally much of the work in relation to placements has been uniprofessional and up to now there has been little sharing of experience and ideas about placements across professions (NHS Executive, 2000). Yet health and social care students come together routinely in placements. There is a need to look at commonality across the professions and to identify transferable issues and solutions regarding pre-registration placements. Before attempting to deliver any form of practice-based interprofessional education, attention should be paid to the process of planning.

It is important to ensure that the aims of joint placement experience are jointly and clearly agreed (Glen, 2001). Miller *et al.* (1999) argue that inexperienced pre-registration students should be offered activities that focus on developing communication skills and understanding one another's professional roles to allow them to develop insights into the concepts that underpin collaboration. Thus a model of interprofessional learning should build on a model of student development. The aims might include:

- Providing students with an understanding of the roles, cultures and values of different professions leading to benefits for patients as a result of increased cooperation and collaboration.
- Facilitating greater confidence by addressing the need sometimes to maintain rigid professional boundaries and identifying the usefulness of the overlap in roles which are different from wasteful duplication.

- Securing a more cost-effective way of providing education and training.
- Contributing to a learning culture, which fosters reflection, analysis and evaluation by focusing on interactive learning.

Prerequisites for success include:

- Identifying common learning outcomes and levels at which they are to be achieved, (QAA, 2001).
- Involving patients as planners, trainers and evaluators (NHS SW Region Office 2002).
- Interprofessional learning groups/sets.
- Using learning and teaching strategies which facilitate interactive teamwork and interprofessional learning. This should include: problem-based learning (PBL) in small mixed groups and joint evaluations (Glen and Wilkie, 2002).
- Identifying a skilled practice facilitator to plan, implement and evaluate the experiences, in addition to drawing out differences, conflicts and commonalities between professional groups (Freeth and Reeves, 1999).
- Common assessments in practice.
- Identifying and planning staff development activities for staff in practice and educational settings (The New Generation Project: www.mhbs.soton.ac.uk/newgeneration).

There is often a wide chasm between academic goals, service requirements and consumer expectations. Clinical governance and National Service Frameworks will be critical in formulating a coherent strategy that satisfies both academic and practice demands. The concept of integrated care pathways provides further opportunities for identifying common ground for both learning and working together, with the ultimate aim of enhancing the quality of care provision. Finally in this section Freeth (2001) makes the very pertinent point that much has been written about promoting interprofessional collaboration in health and social care, but less about ways to sustain it. Many collaborative initiatives are short-lived, ending when initial funds are exhausted, key workers move on, or the management climate becomes less supportive. There is, therefore, very little incentive for stakeholders to publish analyses of terminating collaborations. This is undoubtedly a gap in the current literature (Glen, 2001).

The evolving partnership structures between HEIs and service providers have the potential to raise the profile of practice education and the joint development of academic/practice career pathways.

The development of academic/practice career pathways

Successful partnerships between educators and practising professionals go some way to addressing the integration of theory and practice (Cornes, 1998). Such partnerships provide greater opportunities for lecturers to utilize placements in order to upgrade their knowledge and to familiarize themselves with new technology and trends in client and patient care. The partnership can offer clinical practitioners easier access to the lecturers, who are more conversant with research findings that might have relevance to practice in order to enhance the quality of client and patient care. In addition, lecturers can, through easier access to the placements, have greater opportunities to maintain and develop their own practice expertise. Practice expertise is often difficult for lecturers to maintain (Ioannides, 1999).

A report from the Royal College of Nursing (2001) suggested that pressures from an increasing workload, changes in nursing education and the demands of clinical supervision are damaging morale among nurse lecturers, many of whom feel unable to provide first-class experience for students. The diverse and therefore difficult role in higher education demands theoretical specialization, and an ability to juggle the competing demands of administration, scholarly activity (research and publication), facilitation of learning, academic and pastoral support of students and acting as a link between service and education, especially in relation to clinical supervision of students (Clifford, 1995, Gidman *et al.*, 2000; Haith-Cooper, 1999; Lee, 1996; Murphy, 2000). Ongoing demonstration of practice competence is a cherished hope of educators themselves (Clifford, 1995) but is difficult to accomplish given the multiplicity of roles (see Chapter 1). However, as demonstrated throughout this book, the implementation of *Fitness for Practice* (UKCC, 1999) has created opportunities to reskill lecturers in clinical practice.

Time is universally regarded as the biggest constraint on effective mentoring (Atkins and Williams, 1995; Wilson-Barnett *et al.*, 1995; Watson, 1999; Phillips *et al.*, 2000). Many mentors experience competing demands on their time, and mentoring students often has to give way to the priorities of patient care. Phillips *et al.* (2000) concluded that the validity and reliability of mentors' assessment of students' competence in practice was being compromised by the lack of time that mentors spent working with and observing the student for whom they were responsible. Mentors report giving up their own time to meet their responsibilities towards their students (Atkins and Williams, 1995; Phillips *et al.*, 2000).

The realization that students require support and quality teaching while in practice has emerged as a major issue (Birchenall, 2001). This realization has spawned several new but related jobs, including clinical placement facilitator, practice educator, and clinical facilitator. In terms of practice education, the established role of lecturer practitioner remains the most substantial, particularly as the post-holder can offer expert perspectives from higher education and the practice arena. Much of what facilitators do could be described as bridge building between one element of practice education and another. Theirs is an empowerment role involving the dissemination of good practice across placement areas, troubleshooting where necessary to secure good-quality placements, and also acting as counsellor or mediator when situations become difficult. They act as brokers between HEIs, Confederations and Trusts when deciding on placement areas for particular groups of students. Facilitators also offer support to mentors, particularly where there may be a lack of knowledge surrounding the curriculum.

The Richard Report (CVCP, 1997) and the Smith and Sime (2001) report to the Council of Heads of Medical Schools recognized the importance of developing a practice academic career for medicine and dentistry and the need for higher education, clinical services and the NHS to work together. Unlike in medicine or dentistry, there is no tradition in nursing of academic/practice career pathways (Glen, 2002). This contrasts with the situation in medicine, where academic doctors' involvement in practice is funded via 'SIFT' in England (Service Incremental For Teaching). The Department of Health (2002b) document, *Reforming NHS Education and Training Funds*, provides an opportunity to bring stability to funding arrangements for nursing and allied health profession contracts. This document recommends a fundamental reappraisal of the support for all practice placements and rebasing of funds to distinguish resources supporting learning and development from those supporting service, R&D or other activities. In addition, this document suggests that over time placement support should be redirected to support all healthcare training in the NHS. In particular, placement funding should support teaching activity, common learning during clinical placements, and more multidisciplinary use of clinical teaching facilities.

Differences between salaries and conditions of service between HEIs and the NHS makes transfer between the two systems difficult. Over the last two decades there has emerged a discourse in nurse education relating to the nurse lecturer's involvement in clinical practice (Bendall, 1977; Wong and Wong, 1987; While *et al.*, 1994; Cave, 1994; Wilson-Barnett *et al.*, 1995; May *et al.*, 1997; Runciman *et al.*, 1998). Cave (1994) warned that the teachers of the future will need to maintain their clinical skills to justify their existence. Indeed, the profoundly sensitive question of whether professional educators need to be a separate cadre at all (as opposed to being recruited from practitioners) can no longer be avoided (Glen and Clark, 1999); see also Chapters 1 and 8.

Changes in research and development

There remains a concern about the relative poverty of people within the nursing profession who have the knowledge and experience to undertake rigorous research (DOH, 2000a). The Department of Health (England) published in Autumn 2000 *Towards A Strategy for Nursing and Research* (DOH, 2000). This document represents a significant contribution to developing policy to accelerate the development of the capacity and capability for high-quality nursing research. It also recognizes that nursing's research capacity and capability is compromised by a lack of systematic research training (including management and leadership) attached to salaried posts, as well as the lack of academic/practice career pathways and the fact that practice and research are not well integrated into nursing academic career pathways.

According to the 2001 Research Assessment Exercise (RAE) results published in December 2001, the number of nursing departments that entered the scheme increased from 36 in the last RAE assessment in 1996 to 43. There were 575 staff involved, increased from 397 in the previous exercise. The number of departments with a high rating of 5 increased from one to four, and the number with the lowest rating of 1 dropped from 12 to one. However, no departments were given a top rating of 5* and only six won a rating of 4. More than half of all participating nursing departments were rated 3a or 3b (Lipley, 2002). The report *Research in Nursing and Allied Health Professions* (HEFCE, 2001) maintains that the research base has the potential to deliver improvement provided that there is additional support. The report argues that in the absence of development funding, it is unlikely that it will be economic for HEIs to maintain this improvement to the point where it becomes self-sustaining. However, its main recommendation for delivering improvement is the establishment of a fund to develop and expand the capacity of high-quality research in nursing and allied health professions (AHPs). The purpose of such a fund would be to develop capacity in priority areas not as a primary aim, to fund specific research projects, however, in pursuit of this aim it might support research projects as well as research posts or infrastructure posts.

HEFCE (2002) outlined their response to the recommendations in May. The response stresses the need for a joint Department of Health and HEFCE initiative, and that partners should subsequently include other agencies. An advisory committee has subsequently been set up to include nursing and allied health professions, representation from research councils and charities, and from academics in the field. In addition, the joint DOH/HEFCE personal award scheme, at doctoral and post-doctoral levels, has been launched. It is pertinent to note that the DOH/HEFCE's *Statement of Strategic Alliance for Health and Social Care* (2002a), also previously referred to in this chapter, underlines the DOH's and HEFCE's commitment to share objectives and priorities for research to facilitate joint, strategic and timely plans for the provision of research infrastructure.

There are considerable differences across WDCs with regard to the extent, purpose and manner of the use of Nursing and Midwifery Education and Training Levy (NMET) funding. Research and scholarly activity are essential to support the education of health professionals and thus should be supported from the Education Levy. This view is also supported by the report of the Task Group 3 to HEFCE (2001). The report also argues that the WDCs should be mandated, as a core responsibility, to support research training for teachers in higher education. It also suggests that in the long term confederations should aim to ensure that all lecturers in HE possess research degrees, or have access to the support necessary to acquire them. The HEFCE (2002) response suggests that the current review of all education and training provides a significant opportunity to think afresh about this issue. Possible strategies might include:

- Commissioning of a joint audit, at the national level, between HEIs, the NHS and users and carers to identify the strengths and challenges of existing models, for example: practitioner teachers or lecturer practitioners (Vaughan, 1987), and the establishment of clinical facilitator posts (Birchenall, 2001).

- Commissioning of joint research between HEIs, the NHS and users and carers to clarify types of lecturers, researchers and clinical specialists which might form a bridge between HEIs and the NHS.
- Increased availability of structured training fellowships, which include management and leadership, linked to salaried clinical posts.
- Increased availability of structured and supervised post-doctoral research opportunities with 'academic/practice centres', appropriately funded.
- Protected/dedicated time for practitioners with an education and training remit (for example, mentors and preceptors).
- Infrastructure funding and academic support/link for research active practitioners (Glen and Smith, 1999). Standardization of terms and conditions to facilitate transfer between the NHS and HEIs.
- Identification of a recognized pathway of preparation, qualifications and competencies for the role of lecturer practitioner. (Lathlean, 1997).
- Identification of a funding stream to support nurse lecturers in practice.
- Development of research networks that blur some of the boundaries between practice and academic departments.
- Identification of practice academic career pathways and acknowledgement of the need for extensive flexibility, the aim being to create a range of academic/practice career pathways.
- Ensuring that academics within HEIs remain up to date with developments in the NHS.
- Raising awareness of the healthcare agenda within HEIs by employing senior personnel, for example at Pro Vice-Chancellor level, to liaise with the NHS. This would also promote better dialogue between the NHS and higher education.

The implementation of these recommendations would result in the development of exciting and flexible career pathways for lecturers, researchers and practitioners and contribute to the evolution of a new model of practice education.

Towards a new model of practice education

Nursing education is now clearly part of the higher education sector. The effects of the traditionally all-pervasive ethos of the university might be far-reaching for nursing education and not necessarily beneficial in all instances (Burns and Glen, 2000). The university sector in the twenty-first century is very different from its counterpart in the 1960's and 1970s. The Quality Assurance Agency's endorsement of a learning outcomes approach and identification of the employment-related transferable skills of graduates and postgraduates helps link cognitive attributes with characteristics demonstrated by the responsibility and autonomy of professional work. Fortunately for nursing and allied healthcare professions, the challenges which higher education is having to face – changes in funding mechanisms, the development of lifelong and work-based learning, the increased emphasis on learning outcomes, on graduate capabilities and transferable skills, on students' experience and on employability, as well as the surveillance of research and teaching quality – all facilitate a more flexible model of what it means to be educated (Miers, 2002). What is also needed is a new model of practice education (Glen, 1995). How nurse educators conceptualize needs to change drastically. We need to forge different relationships and partnerships and conceptualize healthcare and experiences of ill-health in new ways.

A cross-disciplinary review by Eraut (1999), which analyses the development of professional knowledge and competence, suggests that for most practice disciplines there is an overemphasis on theory and neglect of structures and opportunities for integrated practical experience for students: 'in spite of increasing evidence that the front loading of theory is extremely inefficient' (p. 12).

Helping students to acquire a sound theoretical knowledge of nursing work and its value is clearly an important aim for pre-registration programmes. However, as emphasized throughout this volume, of equal importance are opportunities to practise skills in order to develop 'know-how', that is, the knowledge of how to do the work of nursing. May *et al.* (1997), for example, refer to one student's awareness of an element of the theory–practice dilemma: 'I know what I should do, I just don't know how to do it.' This would be supported by Schön (1983, p. 16), who argued that although professionals are recognized in society for their professional knowledge, such knowledge does not always enable them to cope with the 'complexity, uncertainty, instability, uniqueness and value conflicts perceived as central to the world of professional practice'.

Pre-1989 models of nurse training, based on apprenticeship models, produced at the point of registration a nurse who had already acquired considerable experience as a member of the nursing workforce and was already perceived by other staff as skilled and experienced. Both the reality of nursing practice and employers' expectations (see Chapter 1) require new nurses to be accountable practitioners at the point of registration. The idea that the pre-registration programme should produce at the moment of registration a skilled and confident practitioner in any setting is still open to question. What it must do is produce, at the point of registration, a practitioner who is safe, competent and supported by a preceptor. The best guarantee of safety is that the practitioner knows the limits of their competence, understands and applies the concept of accountability, recognizes what they cannot do safely, and does not take on tasks or roles for which they will not be competent. Research into the performance and progress of undergraduate nurses has shown that the relevant skills are quickly learned and that within a short time these nurses are at least as skilled as and are more competent than those who have been prepared by the traditional route.

It is timely to acknowledge the importance of clinical education and to redesign pre-registration practice experience to meet both educational and service expectations (Edmond, 2001). This requires that responsibility for, and management of, placements is held at a senior level within an organization. It also requires that a great deal more importance is placed on the role of mentor and preceptor. As Jarvis (1999, p. 272) notes:

> Learning to learn in and from practice needs to form part of the initial curriculum. Practice is the basis not only of our reflective learning, but also the basis on which we construct our own theory. Naturally this involves changing the emphasis in initial preparation and having more teacher/lecturer practitioners, and more mentors and preceptors and placing a great deal more emphasis on their role.

The pivotal issue for the majority of practice areas is that they cannot guarantee availability of staff nurse mentors and preceptors because of heavy workloads; and there is an urgent need to address the issue and to place a great deal more emphasis on their role. Not all mentors are aware of the importance of their role. This may be a legacy from times when students were required to be used as pairs of hands and made up the majority of the clinical team in hospital wards. In many settings this is reflected in the number of placements and the attitudes of many staff who have difficulty recognizing their mentoring role (see Morton-Cooper and Palmer, 1993; Jarvis and Gibson, 1997; Jarvis, 1999; Watson, 1999 Edmond, 2001).

Learning in practice is without doubt a deeply social process that requires time and face-to-face contact (Benner, 1984; Dreyfus, 2001). Benner (1984) studied nurses at each stage of skill acquisition. She found that unless students stay emotionally involved and accepted the joy of a job well done, as well as the remorse of mistakes, they would not develop further and would eventually burn out trying to keep track of all the features and aspects, rules and maxims that modern nursing requires. In general, resistance to involvement and risk leads to stagnation and ultimately to boredom and regression.

The more students are emotionally committed to learning, the better, whereas an expert could be and, indeed, often should be, coldly detached and rational in their practice. This is no doubt true, but the beginner's job is to follow the rules and gain experience, and it is merely a question of motivation whether they are involved or not. Furthermore, the student is not emotionally involved in choosing an action, even if they are involved in its outcomes. Only at the level of competence is there an emotional investment in the choice of action.

Since students tend to imitate mentors, mentors can play a crucial role in whether students withdraw into being disembodied minds or become more and more emotionally involved in the learning situation. If the mentor is detached, the students will be too. Conversely, if the mentor shows their involvement in the way they consider interpretations, is open to students' suggestions and objections, and emotionally dwells on the choices that have led them to their conclusions and actions, the students will be more likely to let their own successes and failures matter to them, and review the choices that led to these outcomes. Only emotional, involved beings can become proficient and expert. So while they are teaching specific skills, mentors must also be role modelling and encouraging involvement. Moreover, learning through apprenticeship requires the presence of experts and being in the presence of more experienced mentors. On this basic level, as Yeats said, 'Man can embody the truth, but he cannot know it.'

The purpose of placement experience should therefore be more than functional task acquisition. Its purpose is well encapsulated in the perspective adopted by Barnard and Dunn (1994), who argue that placement experience should move students beyond simple 'hands-on' tasks; rather, students 'need to engage their compassion, thoughts and judgements in all experiences' (Barnard and Dunn, 1994). Practice requires integration of thinking, feeling and doing. Learning and participation is also not simply a way of acquiring skills, but also of developing an identity and sense of belonging in the community. The activities in which students participate will construct meaning and reality for them. Thus a mentor working with students must be aware of their impact, as role models, on students' learning and self-efficiency expectations. In essence the quality of those who provide a role model will dictate the quality of the nurses produced (Theobald, 1995).

Early guided immersion in the reality of practice should also encourage development of social and corporate responsibility and a sense of belonging, as well as personal professional development (UKCC, 1999; Eraut, 1990). Students often complain of feeling alienated from the nursing team and affected by the negative attitude of some staff towards them (Bain, 2001). However, involvement in pre-registration education is widely seen as a benefit for clinical staff for their continuing professional development and for clinical governance (NHS Executive, 2000). Part of the problem has been identified as the misunderstanding or misinterpretation of the term 'supernumerary status'. Joyce (1999) outlines a framework for implementing supernumerary learning in a pre-registration programme, with the mentor playing a vital role. During students' initial stages of observation, the mentors take on an active, leading role. As the students progress towards a more participatory stage, mentors take the role of a catalyst guiding students through the experience. Mentors' roles change as students continue to progress with the placement, becoming less 'directive' and more of a moderator, encouraging reflection and self-directed learning.

The evidence is that because clinical skills are context dependent, and the ability to apply knowledge and perform competently depends on familiarity with the specific clinical context, this can be achieved more easily where there is initial close linking between the mentor and the student, and optimizing of learning opportunities (Steinaker and Bell, 1979; Benner, 1984; Hinchliff, 1992; Davies *et al.*, 1999; Edmond, 2001). It also relates to the perceptual wholeness of interactive learning opportunities and situated cognition, which claims that learning is occurring with every human behaviour and that human knowledge is located in physical interaction and social participation (Clancy, 1997; Lave and Wenger, 1991). It would be timely to debate the following key questions:

- How many different placements must students experience in order to achieve the competence and fitness to practice?
- What is the purpose of students' placements?
- To what extent is it feasible for students to learn by attachments to patients/service users and their care pathways?

A theoretical perspective that sheds light on the learning process in placements is described as learning that is situated in social practice. Lave and Wenger (1991) offer an analysis of learning which takes as its focus the relationship between learning and the social situations in which it occurs. It differs most radically from other perspectives in that the focus of learning, rather than being situated in the individual mind, takes place within a framework of social participation (Elkjaer, 1999). Lave and Wenger (1991) adopt the term 'situated learning' to explain this learning in action that occurs through social performance. This, they propose is a concept that attempts to take as its focus not simply a geographical perspective, for example, a student learning in a particular location, but the nature of the relationship between the learning that occurs and the social situation (Hanks, 1991). Therefore, the success of any approach to practical education depends on tackling the major problem of availability of mentors or clinical educators and provision of appropriate structures and resources to ensure that they have the time, the tools and the training to provide quality practical education and experience.

Conclusion

A collaborative approach is capable of addressing the intellectual challenge of developing a new paradigm of practice. The concept and practice of professional education needs to be developed into a more rigorous discipline and, therefore, needs a well-integrated and powerful collaborative team approach. Such aspirations can easily be lost in the struggle for dwindling resources. Funding for dedicated time in education for practice staff and dedicated time in practice for lecturers is a vital and pivotal issue, and one that has crippled past efforts to ensure support and quality guidance for both pre-registration and newly qualified nurses. The identification of such a funding stream would greatly facilitate the further development and evaluation of the practice-based learning and teaching models outlined in the previous chapters, in addition to the development of integrated clinical academic career pathways in nursing. Given the necessary funding and incentives, there is no doubt that collaborative partnerships between HEIs and service and across professions could be predicated to facilitate the development and implementation of models of nursing education capable of recognizing the primacy of professional practice.

Finally, robust health and education sector partnerships and networks across health economics would support the modernization of the NHS, with thriving research, learning, knowledge management and education and service relationships across organizational boundaries, through:

- effective joint strategic planning; and
- effective joint working within and between the sectors.

Strategic Health Authorities, Workforce Development Confederations, Primary Care Trusts and Higher Education Institutions have a key role to play in the development of local Health and Education Sector Partnerships (Pearson, 2002). At the heart of such changes is the public, and students supported by the HEI – service partnership.

References

Atkins, S and Williams, A (1995) Registered Nurses' Experiences of Mentoring Undergraduate Nursing Students, *Journal of Advanced Nursing*, **21**(5), 1006–15.

Bain, D (2001) 'Social Learning Theory: Its Application In the Context of Nurse Education', *Nurse Education Today*, **21**(2), 83–155.

Barnard, P and Dunn, D (1994) 'Issues in The Organisation and Structure from Clinical Education for Undergraduate Nursing Programmes', *Journal of Nursing Education*, **33**(90), 420–2.

Barr, H (2001) *Interprofessional Education: Tensions and Contradictions?* St Bartholomew School of Nursing and Midwifery, Second Annual Lecture, 7 March 2001. Available from S. Glen, St Bartholomew School of Nursing and Midwifery, City University, London EC1A 7QN.

Bendall, E (1977) The Future of British Nurse Education, *Journal of Advanced Nursing*, **2**(2), 171–81.

Benner, P (1984) *From Novice to Expert: Excellence and Power in Clinical Nursing Practice*. Menlo Park, CA: Addison-Wesley.

Birchenall, P (2001) 'Education Facilitation : A Developing Role', *Nurse Education Today* **21**, 249–50.

Breckenridge, A (2002) *Future Direction in Higher Education: What will the Relationship Between Universities and the NHS Look Like in Five Year's Time?* HEFCE, Universities UK and Nuffield Trust Seminar, London, 8 March 2002. www.universitiesuk.ac.uk/healtheducation.

Burns, I and Glen, S (2000) An Educational Model for Preparation for Practice. In Glen, S and Burns, I, *Problem Based Learning in Nursing: A New Model for a New Context?* Basingstoke, Macmillan – now Palgrave Macmillan.

Cable, S (2000) Clinical Experience: Preparation of Medical and Nursing Students for Collaborative Practices. Unpublished PhD thesis, University of Dundee, December.

Cave, I (1994) Nurse Teachers in Higher Education – without clinical competence – do they have a future?, *Nurse Education Today*, **14**, 394–9.

Clancy, W J (1997) *Situated Cognition on Human Knowledge and Computer Representations.* Cambridge: Cambridge University Press.

Clifford, C (1995) The Role of the Nurse Teacher: Concerns, Conflicts and Challenges, *Nurse Education Today*, **15**, 11–16.

Committee of Vice-Chancellors and Principals (1997) *Clinical Academic Careers: Report of An Independent Task Force.* Chaired by Professor Rex Richard.

Corbett, K (1998) The Captive Market in Nurse Education and the Displacement of Nursing Knowledge, *Journal of Advanced Nursing*, **28**(3), 524–31.

Cornes, D (1998) Some Thoughts on Nurse Education Service Partnerships, *Nurse Education Today*, **18**, 655.

Davies, E, Turner, C and Osborne, Y (1999) Evaluating a Clinical Partnership Model for Undergraduate Nurse Students, *Collegian* **6**, 23–40.

Department of Health (1999) *Making a Difference: Strengthening the Nursing, Midwifery and Health Visiting Contribution to Health and Healthcare.* London: DOH.

Department of Health (2000) *Towards A Strategy for Nursing and Research.* London: DOH.

Department of Health (2000a) *Consultative Document: A Health Service Of All The Talents: Developing The N.H.S. Workforce.* London: DOH.

Department of Health (2000b) *The NHS Plan: A Plan For Investment: A Plan For Reform.* London: DOH.

Department of Health (2001a) *Working Together, Learning Together: A Framework for Lifelong Learning in the NHS.* London: DOH.

Department of Health (2001b) *Shifting the balance of power within the NHS: securing delivery.* London: DOH.

Department of Health (2002b) *Reforming NHS Education and Training Funds.* London: DOH (MLD/28).

Department of Health and the Higher Education Funding Council for England (2002a), *Statement of Strategic Alliance for Health and Social Care.* London: DOH.

Dreyfus, H L (2001) *On The Internet: Thinking in Action,* London: Routledge.

Edmond, C (2001) A New Paradigm for Practice Education, *Nurse Education Today*, **21**, 251–9.

Elkjaer, B (1999) In Search of Social Learning Theory. In Easterby-Smith, M, Burgoyne, J and Araugo, H (eds), *'Organisational Learning' and the Learning Organisation.* London: Sage.

Eraut, M (1999) *Developing Professional Knowledge and Competence*, 4th edn. London: The Falmer Press.

Freeth, D (2001) Sustaining Interprofessional Collaboration, *Journal of Interprofessional Care*, **15**(1), 37–46.

Freeth, D and Reeves, S (1999) *Interprofessional Training Ward Pilot Phase: Evaluation Project Report.* St Bartholomew School of Nursing and Midwifery, City University, Internal Research Report, Number 19.

Gidman, J, Humphreys, A and Andrews, M (2000) The Role of The Personal Tutor in the Academic Context, *Nurse Education Today*, **20**, 401–7.

Glen, S (1995) Towards A New Model of Nursing Education, *Nurse Education Today*, **15**, 90–5.

Glen, S (2000) Partnerships: The Way Forward, *Nurse Education Today*, **20**, 339–40.

Glen, S (2001) Transdisciplinary Education: Tensions and Contradictions?, *Nursing Times Research*, **6**(5), 2–11.

Glen, S (2002) The Creation of Roles Straddling Academia and Practice, *Learning in Health and Social Care*, No. 1, 59–66.

Glen, S and Clark, A (1999) Nurse Education: A Skill Mix for the Future, *Nurse Education Today*, **19**, 12–19.

Glen, S and Smith, K (1999) Towards New Models of Teaching and Researching Nursing: The Research Practitioner, *Nurse Education Today*, **19**, 628–32.

Glen, S and Wilkie, K (2002) *Problem–based Learning in Nursing : A New Model for a New Context?* 2nd edn. Basingstoke: Palgrave Macmillan.

Haith-Cooper, M (2000) Problem Based Learning Within Health Professional Education. What Is The Role Of The Lecturer? A Review of the Literature, *Nurse Education Today*, **20**, 267–72.

Hanks, W (1991) Foreword. In Lave, J and Wenger, E (eds), *Situated Learning: Legitimate Peripheral Participation*, Cambridge: Cambridge University Press.

Higher Education Funding Council for Education (2001) *Research in Nursing and Allied Health Professions*. Bristol, November (Report 01.63).

Higher Education Funding Council for Education (2002) *Research Capacity in Nursing and Allied Health Professions: Joint Response by the Department of Health and HEFCE to the Recommendations of the Task Group 3 Report*. Bristol, HEFCE, May (circular letter no. 10/02).

Hinchliff, S (ed). *The Practitioner As Teacher*. London: Scutari Press.

Ioannides, A (1999) The Nurse Teacher's Clinical Role Now and In The Future, *Nurse Education Today*, (1999) **19**, 207–14.

Jarvis, P (1999) The Way Forward For Practice Education, *Nurse Education Today*, **19**, 269–73.

Jarvis, P and Gibson, S (1997) *The Teacher Practitioner and Mentor in Nursing Hesalth Visiting, Midwifery and Social Work*, 2nd edn. Cheltenham: Nelson Thornes.

Joyce, P (1999) Implementing Supernumerary Learning In A Pre-Registration Diploma in Nursing Programme : An Action Research Study, *Journal of Clinical Nursing*, **8**(5), 567–76.

Koppel, I, Barr, H, Reeves, S, Freeth, D and Hammick, M, (2001) Establishing A Systematic Approach To evaluating The Effectiveness of Interprofessional Education, *Issues in Interdisciplinary Care*, **3**, 41–9.

Lave, J and Wenger, E, (1991) *Situated Learning: Legitimate Peripheral Participation*. Cambridge: Cambridge University Press.

Lathlean, J (1997) *Lecture Practitioners in Action.* Guildford: Butterworth–Heinemann.

Lee, DTF (1996) The Clinical Role Of The Nurse Teacher : A Review of The Dispute, *Journal of Advanced Nursing*, **23**, 1127–34.

Lipley, N (2002) Could Do Better, *Nursing Standard*, 3 January.

May, N, Vetch, L, McIntosh, J and Alexander, M (1997) *Preparation for Practice: Evaluation of Nurse and Midwife Education in Scotland, 1992 Programmes.* Final Report, Edinburgh: NBS.

Miers, M (2002) Nurse Education in Higher Education: Understanding Cultural Barriers to Progress, *Nurse Education Today*, **22**, 212–19.

Miller, C, Ross, N and Freeman, N (1999) *Shared Learning and Clinical Teamwork: new directions in education for multiprofessional practice.* London. ENB.

Morton-Cooper, A and Palmer, A (1993) *Mentoring and Preceptorship: A Guide To Support Roles In Clinical Practice.* London: Blackwell Scientific Publications.

Murphy, F (2000) Collaborating With Practitioners In Teaching and Research: A Model For Developing The Role of The Nurse Lecturer in Practice Areas, *Journal of Advanced Nursing*, **31**(3), 704–14.

National Audit Office Report (2001) *Educating and Training The Future Health Professional Workforce for England.* London: NAO.

NHS Executive (2000) *Clinical Placements in Primary and Community Care Projects*, June.

NHS South West Regional Office (2002) *Learning and Working Together.* NHS South West Regional Office.

Pearson, M (2002) *Health and education Sector Partnerships (HESPs) Briefing for Strategic Health Authority Chief Executives.* DOH, 7 January.

Phillips, T, Shostak, J, Tyler, J and Allen, L (2000) *Practice and Assessment: An Evaluation of the assessment of practice at diploma degree and postgraduate level in pre and post registration nursing and midwifery education.* English National Board Research Highlight No. 43.

QAA (2001) *Benchmarking Academic and Practitioner Standards in Health Care Subjects.* Bristol: Quality Assurance Agency for Higher Education.

Royal College of Nursing (2001) Workload Pressure on Nurse Lecturers in Higher Education Is Damaging, *Nurse Education*, London: RCN.

Royal College of Nursing (2002) Nursing Education: A Statement of Principles, *Nurse Education*, London: RCN.

Runciman P, Dewar, B and Goulbourne, A (1998) *Project 2000 in Scotland: Employers' Needs and the Skills of Newly Qualified Project 2000 Staff Nurses.* Edinburgh National Board for Nursing, Midwifery and Health Visiting for Scotland.

Schön, D A (1983) *The Reflective Practitioner: How Professionals Think in Action.* Aldershot: Arena.

Smith, T and Sime, T (2001) *A Survey of Clinical Academic Staffing Levels in UK Medical and Dental Schools.* A Report to the Council of Heads of Medical Schools and Deans of UK Faculties of Medicine.

Steinaker, N and Bell, R (1979) *The Experiential Taxonomy: A new approach to Teaching and Learning.* London: Academic Press.

The Learning and Teaching Support Network for Health Sciences and Practice (2002), *Interprofessional Education Today, Yesterday and Tomorrow: A Review.*

Theobald, M (1995) Nursing Must First Become A Profession of Graduates, *British Journal of Nursing,* **5**(1), 6–7.

Tope, R (1996) *Interdisciplinary Learning Between The Health and Social Care Professions: A Feasibility Study.* Aldershot: Avebury.

UKCC (1994), *A Statement of Strategic Intent.* London: UKCC.

UKCC (1999), *Fitness for Practice,* The UKCC Commission for Nursing and Midwifery Education chaired by Sir Leonard Peach. London: UKCC.

Vaughan, B (1987) Bridging The Gap, *Senior Nurse,* **6**(5), 30–3.

Watson, N A (1999) Mentoring today – the students' views. An investigative case study of pre-registration nursing students' experiences and perceptions of mentoring on one theory/practice module of the Common Foundation Programme on a Project 2000 Course, *Journal of Advanced Nursing,* **29**(1), 254–62.

While, E *et al.* (1994) *A Detailed Study of the Relationship between Teaching, Support, Supervision and Role Modelling in Clinical Areas within the Context of Project 2000 Courses.* London: ENB.

Wilson-Barnett, J *et al.* (1995) Clinical Support and the Project 2000 Nursing Students – Factors Influencing the Process, *Journal of Advanced Nursing,* **21**, 1152–8.

Wong, J and Wong, S (1987) Towards Effective Clinical Teaching in Nursing, *Journal of Advanced Nursing,* **12**(4), 505–10.

Zwarenstein, M, Atkins, J, Barr, H, Hammick, M, Koppel, I and Reeves, S (1999) A Systematic Review of Interprofessional Education, *Journal of Interprofessional Care,* **13**(4), 417–24.

Useful Web Addresses

Centre for Health Sciences and Practice
www.health.ltsn.ac.uk

The New Generation Project: Taking Forward Common Learning in Health Professional Education
www.mhbs.soton.ac.uk/newgeneration

UK Centre for the Advancement of Interprofessional Education (CAIPE)
www.caipe.org.uk

Index